PATHOGNOMIA

THE VISUAL LANGUAGE OF CLINICAL SIGNS

DR GAURANG SAMANT
DR PRIYA JHA
DR ASHWINI RANI SR

Clever Fox® PUBLISHING
Chennai • Bangalore

CLEVER FOX PUBLISHING
Chennai, India

Published by CLEVER FOX PUBLISHING 2026

ISBN: 978-93-7500-447-9

"All you need is a little delusion and audacity, and you can seriously do anything in this world".

– Alex Goldie

Dedicated to

Our Parents for their unconditional love and support.

FOREWORD

In the evolving landscape of medical education, the ability to retain key clinical signs is vital for efficient diagnosis and patient care. *Pathognomia* breaks away from traditional rote learning by presenting pathognomonic signs in a format that is both educational and engaging.

Dr. Gaurang Samant, Dr. Priya Jha, and Dr. Ashwini Rani SR have created a work that fuses core clinical concepts with an added touch of humor. This book not only serves as a compact reference but also as a visual toolkit for students, interns, and practitioners revisiting classic signs.

I commend the authors for their innovative approach and hope *Pathognomia* becomes a staple in clinical learning libraries across campuses.

Dr Shashikiran N D,
Dean, School of Dental Sciences, KVV

PREFACE

The spark for *Pathognomia* came from a simple yet persistent struggle during our clinical years, remembering rare but essential clinical signs. We found ourselves scribbling cartoons, making memes, and crafting humorous analogies just to remember that Auspitz's sign had "pinpoint bleeding" or that the "Soap Bubble" appearance wasn't about hygiene but about radiology.

So, we thought, why not compile all of this into a visually rich, clinically relevant handbook? *Pathognomia* is a product of that idea, caffeine- fueled nights, and shared ambition.

This book is for every student who has ever panicked before rounds, every friend who asked, "Is there a trick to remember this?" and every teacher who made signs stick with a story.

We hope it helps you the way it helped us, with a smile and a solid diagnosis.

With warm hearts and tired brains,

Dr. Gaurang Samant

Dr. Priya Jha

Dr. Ashwini Rani SR

AUTHORS DETAILS

Dr. Gaurang Ashwin Samant and **Dr. Priya Bipin Jha,** graduates of the BDS program at the School of Dental Sciences, Karad, share a commitment to making medical and dental learning clearer, faster, and more engaging for students.

Dr. Gaurang Ashwin Samant has a strong interest in clinical diagnostics and in simplifying complex concepts for better recall. Beyond academics, he is passionate about theatre, drama, and modern cinema, and enjoys exploring diverse cuisines. His appreciation for pure coffee and his creative outlook contributes to the distinct learning style reflected in this book.

Dr. Priya Bipin Jha has navigated the demanding balance of clinics, textbooks, and deadlines. Her love for travel-mountains, snowfall, and local food-remains a constant aspiration. She values simple, grounding moments with friends and peaceful evenings by the sea, where she reflects and unwinds. Her thoughtful, observant nature complements her dedication as a clinician.

Dr Ashwini Rani SR. Associate Professor, finished BDS in the year 2000 and MDS in the year 2011 under RGUHS, presently working in Krishna Vishwa Vidyapeeth for 14 years with 82 national and international publications .65 copyrights, six patents and five text book chapters has contribution to the field of Oral Medicine & Radiology.

OBJECTIVES

- To simplify the understanding of pathognomonic signs by providing clear, concise, and clinically relevant descriptions tailored to dental and medical students.
- To enhance memory retention of important diagnostic signs through visual aids, humor, and meme-based illustrations.
- To create a quick-reference clinical guide that can be used during ward rounds, viva prep, case discussions, and entrance exam revision.
- To encourage integrated learning by combining history, pathophysiology, clinical presentation, and treatment aspects of each sign.
- To bridge the gap between theory and bedside application by helping learners connect textbook knowledge with real-life clinical clues.
- To foster active recall and visual learning, especially for signs that are less commonly encountered but high-yield in diagnosis.
- To cultivate diagnostic curiosity and pattern recognition among undergraduates, interns, and postgraduates in clinical settings.

INDEX

SECTION I

DERMATOLOGICAL & MUCOCUTANEOUS SIGNS

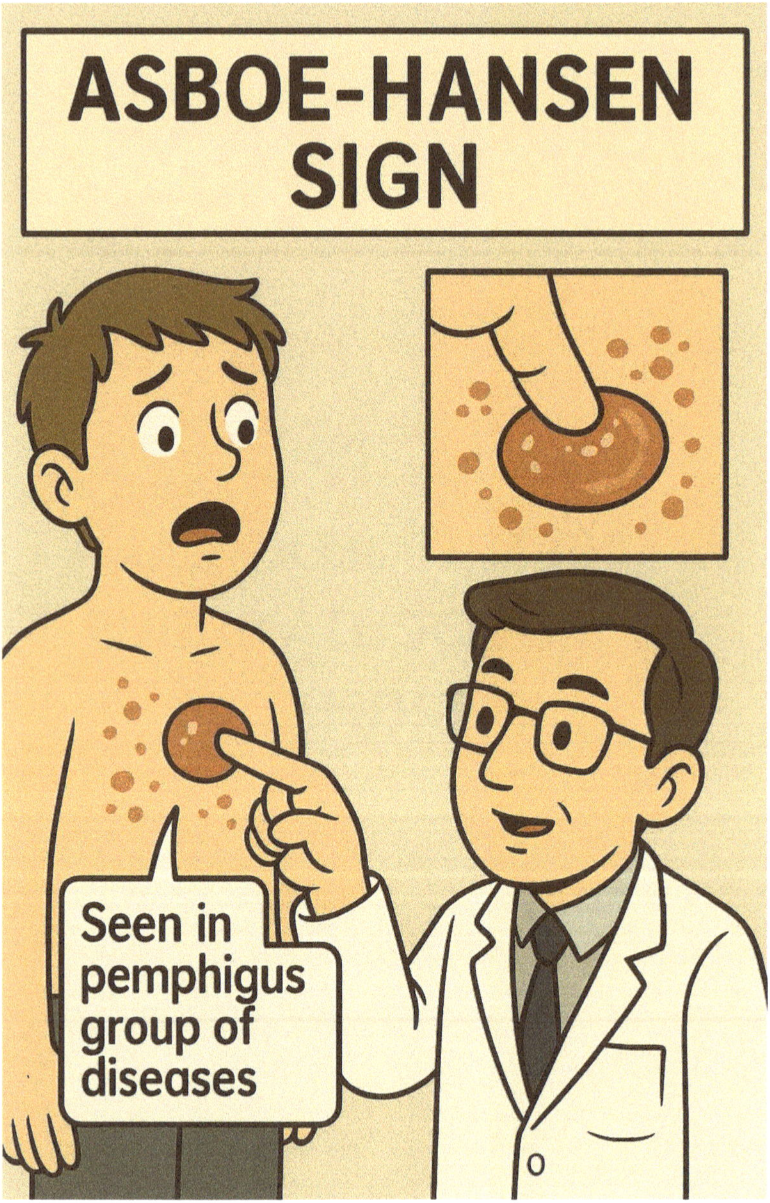
ASBOE-HANSEN SIGN
Seen in pemphigus group of diseases

Asboe-Hansen Sign

- **Name given after** Sir Gustav Asboe-Hansen.
- **Other names:** - Indirect Nikolsky sign, Nikolsky II sign, Bulla Spread sign.
- **Denotes** to the spread of blister to the neighboring unblistered skin when pressure is applied on the top of the bulla.
- It is positive when elicited in all varieties of blistering diseases like:
    - Pemphigus group of diseases
    - Many cases of subepidermal blisters including:
        1. Bullous pemphigoid.
        2. Dermatitis herpetiformis.
        3. Dystrophic epidermolysis bullosa.
        4. Bullous drug eruptions.
        5. Acute bullous lichen planus.

TREATMENT

Category	Details
Goals of Treatment	Suppress autoantibody production, Promote lesion healing, Minimize long-term corticosteroid side effects Hospitalization for all but minor cases.

Initial Management	Wound care similar to partial-thickness burns: • Reverse isolation • Hydrocolloid or silver sulfadiazine dressings
Mild Disease	**First-line:** Rituximab or Prednisone (0.5–1 mg/kg/day) ± Azathioprine or Mycophenolate mofetil
Moderate to Severe Disease	Rituximab + Prednisone (1–1.5 mg/kg/day)± Azathioprine or Mycophenolate mofetil- IV methylprednisolone pulse (1 g/day) may be used
Adjunctive Therapies	**Immunosuppressants:** Rituximab Azathioprine Mycophenolate mofetil **Plasma exchange** or **IVIG** to lower autoantibody titters.
Referral	- To a dermatologist with pemphigus expertise

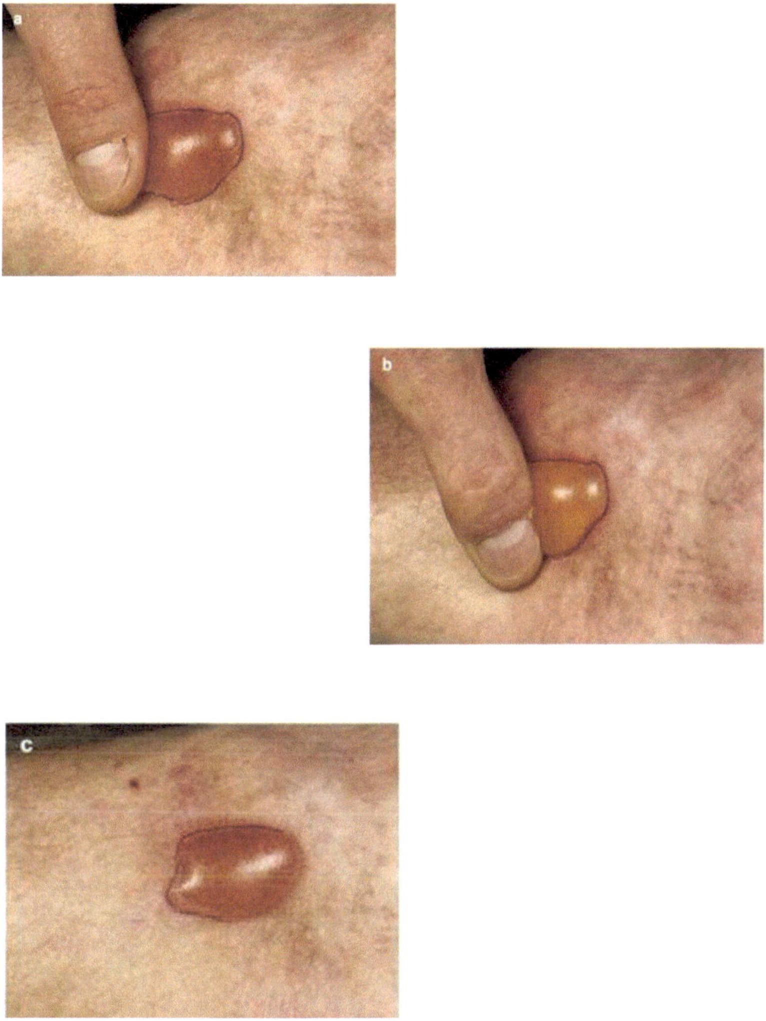

Jonkman, M.F., Horváth, B. (2022). Dermatological Examination of Bullous Diseases. In: Horváth, B. (eds) Autoimmune Bullous Diseases. Springer, Cham.

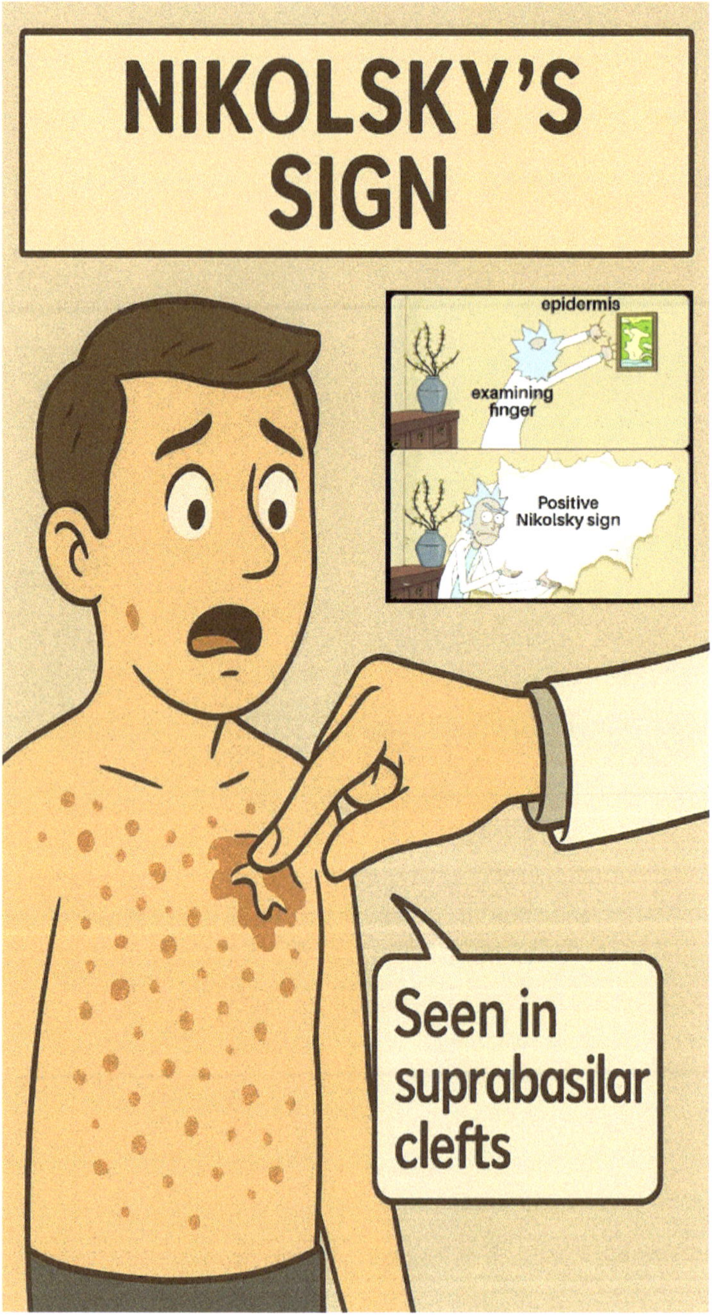
NIKOLSKY'S SIGN
epidermis
examining finger
Positive Nikolsky sign
Seen in suprabasilar clefts

Nikolsky's Sign

- **First described by** Dr. Pyotr Vasilyewich Nikolsky in the year 1896.
- **Pathognomic for:**
  - Pemphigus
  - Toxic epidermal necrolysis
  - Staphylococcal scalded skin syndrome (SSSS)
- **Differentiates** intraepidermal blisters from subepidermal blisters.
- **Induced by** applying lateral or tangential pressure with a thumb or finger to the surrounding skin, the affected area or even apparently healthy skin, which generates a force that separates the upper layers of the epidermis from the lower layers.
- **Types:**
  1. **Wet Nikolsky's sign**: - The base appears moist, shiny, and worn away.
  2. **Dry Nikolsky's sign**: - The base of the damaged skin is dry.
  3. **Marginal Nikolsky's sign**: - Erosion spreads into the adjacent healthy skin.
  4. **Direct Nikolsky's sign**: - Erosion is induced on normal skin situated far from the lesions.
  5. **False Nikolsky's sign**: - Also known as Sheklakov's sign, this sign occurs when pulling the outer edge of a ruptured blister, thereby spreading erosion into the nearby healthy skin.
  6. **Pseudo Nikolsky's sign**: - The underlying mechanism involves necrosis rather than acantholysis.

TREATMENT

Condition	Treatment
Pemphigus vulgaris	• Systemic corticosteroids (e.g., Prednisolone) • Immunosuppressants (Azathioprine, Mycophenolate mofetil) • Rituximab (biologic) • Supportive care (wound care, fluids)
Stevens–Johnson Syndrome (SJS) /Toxic Epidermal Necrolysis (TEN)	• Immediate withdrawal of the causative drug • ICU or burn unit care - IV fluids, electrolyte management • Pain control, wound care - IVIG or cyclosporine (optional)
Staphylococcal Scalded Skin Syndrome (SSSS)	• IV antibiotics (e.g., Nafcillin, Oxacillin, Vancomycin if MRSA) • Supportive care (fluids, wound care)
Pemphigus foliaceus	• Similar to pemphigus vulgaris: corticosteroids + immunosuppressants

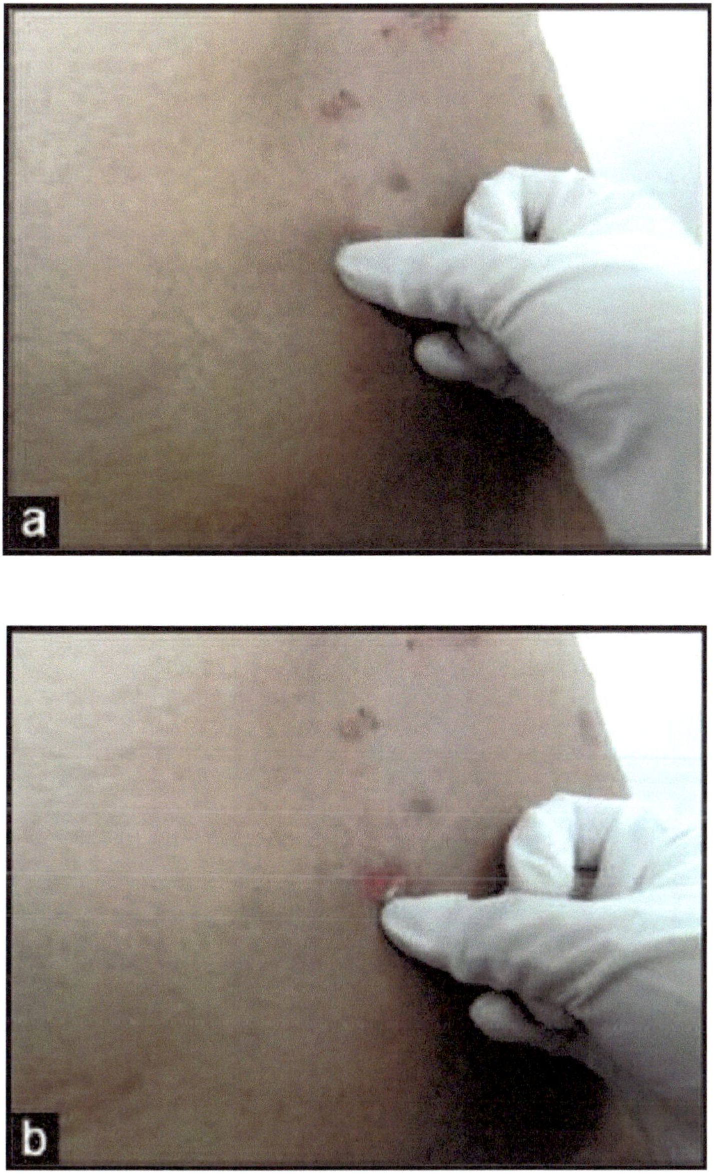

Seshadri, Divya & Kumaran, Muthu Sendhil & Kanwar, Amrinder. (2013). Acantholysis revisited: Back to basics. Indian journal of dermatology, venereology and leprology. 79. 120-6. 10.4103/0378-6323.104688.

WHEN YOU RUB A SUSPICIOUS SKIN LESION...

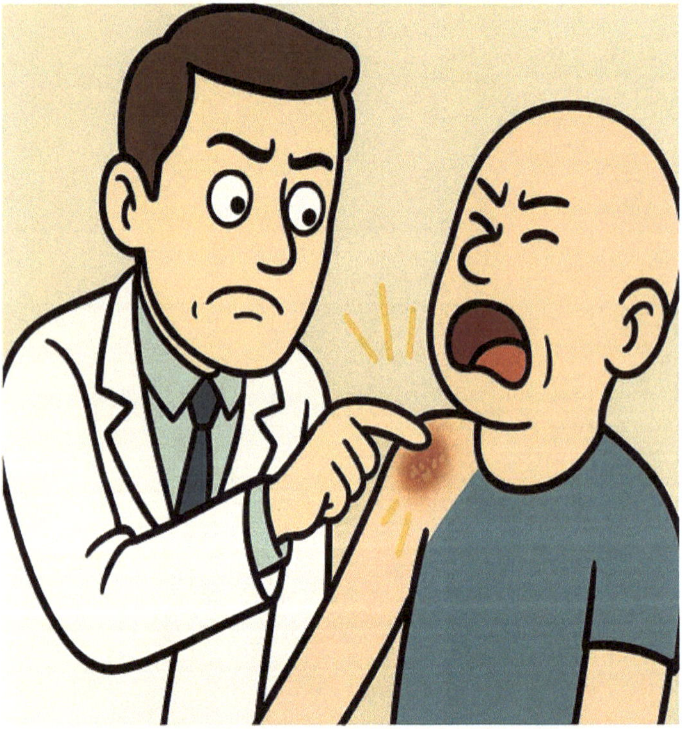

AND IT FLARES UP IN RESPONSE

Darier's Sign

- Darier's sign is a dermatological reaction characterized by the appearance of a wheal and flare (redness and swelling) after stroking or rubbing a skin lesion. This sign is particularly associated with cutaneous Masto cytosis and urticaria pigmentosa, where it indicates the release of mast cell mediators like histamine.

- **What it looks like:**
  - ➢ When a lesion on the skin of someone with Masto cytosis is gently rubbed or stroked, it typically will become red, itchy, and swollen (wheal and flare) within a few minutes.

- **What causes it:**
  - ➢ This reaction is due to mast-cell degranulation in the skin, which releases histamine and other mediators into the surrounding tissue.

- **Clinical significance:**
  - ➢ A positive Darier's sign is a key diagnostic feature of Masto cytosis and urticaria pigmentosa, helping to differentiate these conditions from other skin conditions.

- **How it's elicited:**
  - ➢ The symptom can be induced by stroking the lesion with a blunt instrument, such as a tongue depressor or a fingernail.

- **Differentiation from other conditions:**
  - Darier's sign helps distinguish Masto cytosis from other conditions that might present with similar skin lesions, such as psoriasis or some types of dermatitis.

TREATMENT

Category	Treatment Options
General Measures	• Avoid triggers: sun, heat, sweating • Gentle skin care: avoid harsh soaps and scrubbing
Topical Treatments	• **Retinoids:** Isotretinoin, tazarotene, adapalene (reduce hyperkeratosis) • **Fluorouracil (5-FU):** Inhibits DNA synthesis • **Corticosteroids:** Reduce inflammation and itching
Oral Treatments	• **Oral retinoids:** Acitretin, isotretinoin for severe cases • **Other systemic meds:** Cyclosporine, dupilumab (under investigation)
Local Treatments	• **Surgical excision:** For localized hypertrophic lesions • **Photodynamic therapy:** Targets abnormal skin cells

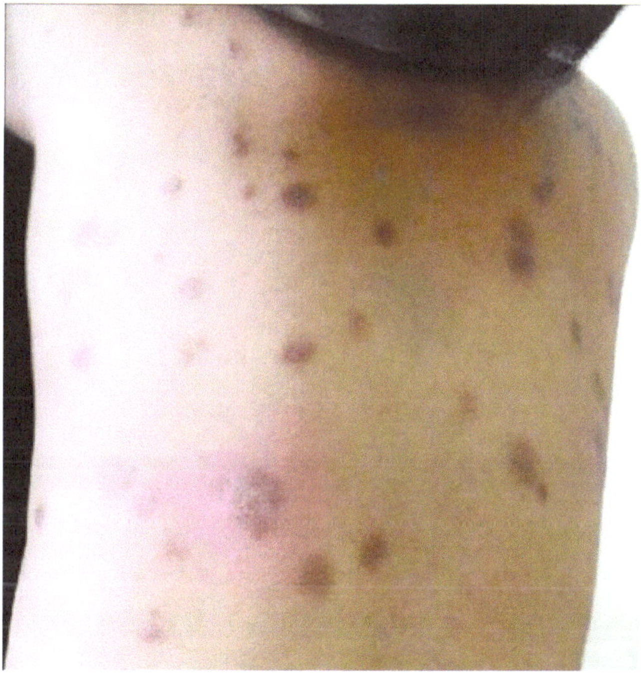

Srinivas, Sahana. (2015). Mastocytosis in children.

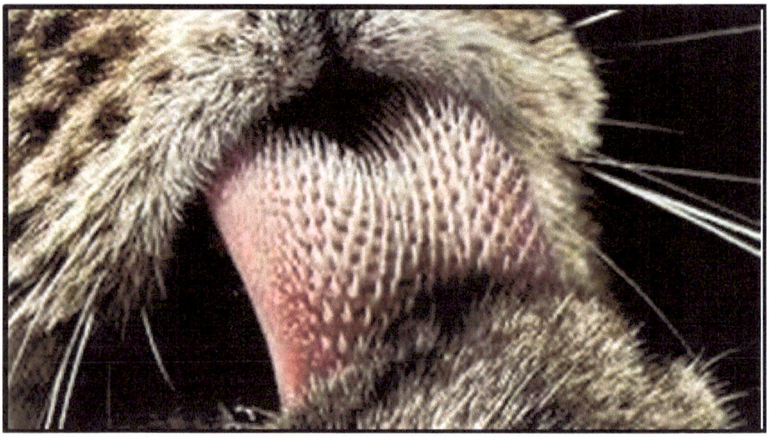

Carpet Tack Sign

- The "carpet tack sign" in dermatology is a visible sign of adherent scales in hair follicles, resembling the undersurface of a perforated carpet or a carpet tack.
- It's often associated with Discoid Lupus Erythematosus (DLE).
- The sign is also known as "Tin-Tack Sign" or "Cat's Tongue Sign".

- **Formation:**
  - ➢ Scales accumulate within individual hair follicles, leading to a characteristic appearance.

- **Appearance:**
  - ➢ When scales are removed, the underlying follicular structures (like the "tacks" of a carpet tack) become visible, creating the "carpet tack sign".

- **Significance:**
  - ➢ While the sign is commonly associated with DLE, it can also be seen in other conditions like seborrheic dermatitis and pemphigus foliaceous, but in DLE, bleeding may occur after scale removal.

TREATMENT

Category	Measures
General Measures	• Year-round sun protection (clothing + high SPF sunscreen) • Avoid glass windows or use UV-blocking films • Vitamin D supplements (if sun avoided) • Smoking cessation
Local Therapy	• Potent/ultrapotent topical corticosteroids (intermittent courses) • Intralesional corticosteroid injections • Calcineurin inhibitors (tacrolimus, pimecrolimus) • Cosmetic camouflage and wigs for scarring
Systemic Therapy	• Short-term: Prednisone or prednisolone • Long-term options Hydroxychloroquine, chloroquine, oral retinoids (isotretinoin, acitretin) Mycophenolate mofetil, ciclosporin, cyclophosphamide • Azathioprine, dapsone, thalidomide

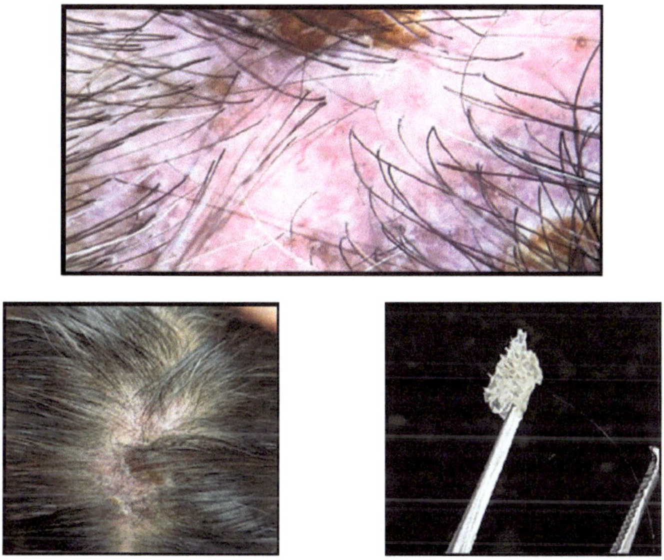

Mitra D, Bhatnagar A, Sanoj PK, Singh A. Bedside Dermoscopy and Demonstration of Tin-tack Sign in Discoid Lupus Erythematosus. Indian J Postgrad Dermatol. 2024;2:50-1. doi: 10.25259/IJPGD_83_2023

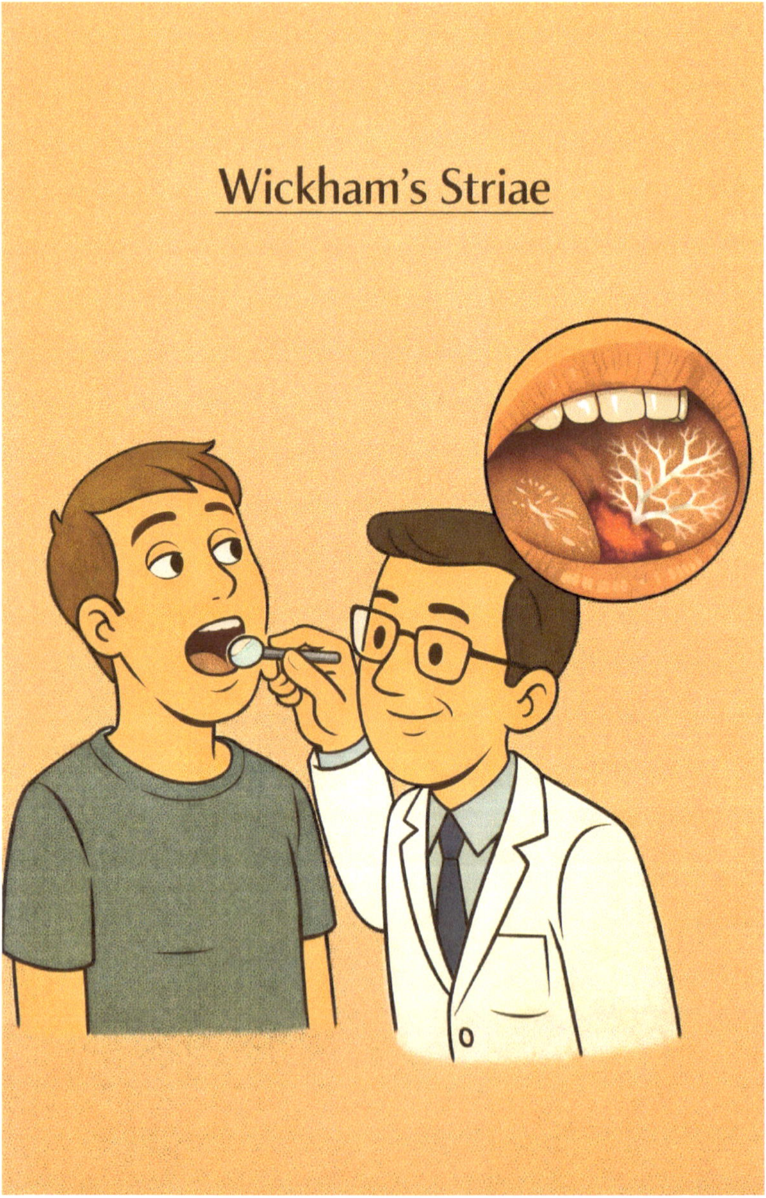
Wickham's Striae

Wickham's Striae

- First coined by Louis Frédéric Wickham in the year 1895.
- The presence of fine white or grayish lines or dots is observed on the surface of the papular rash and mucosal lesions associated with Lichen planus.
- Within the oral cavity, these lesions often display tree-like patterns or a lacy network appearance, typically presenting bilaterally and more commonly found on the buccal mucosa.
- They may also occur on the lateral edges of the tongue, gums, and lips.

Pathogenesis:

1. Darier *et al.*	Attributes the appearance of the Wickham's striae (WS) to an increase in the granular cell layer of the epidermis.
2. Summerly *et al.*	Gave the explanation of focal increase in epidermal activity leading to the formation of striae.
3. Ryan	Suggested a pathological factor for the formation of WS: a lack of dermal vessels in the area which acts as a contributing factor

- Histological confirmation of WS can be performed using India ink staining, which highlights ink retention in the stratum corneum.

TREATMENT

Type	Measure/Treatment	Details
General Care	Avoid harsh soaps/ gels Emollients	Prevents scaling Maintain hydration Reduce night- time itch
Topical Therapy	Sedating antihistamines Potent corticosteroids Calcineurin inhibitors Retinoids	Creams or steroid tape Tacrolimus, Pimecrolimus Topical vitamin A derivatives For localized lesions
Systemic Therapy	Intralesional steroids Oral steroids Immunosuppressants Others Phototherapy	Short course (1– 3 months) Methotrexate, Azathioprine, Mycophenolate Acitretin, Hydroxychloroq uine NB-UVB/PUVA (not for actinicus)
Other Options	Antibiotics/ Antifungals	Metronidazole, Sulfasalazine, Griseofulvin

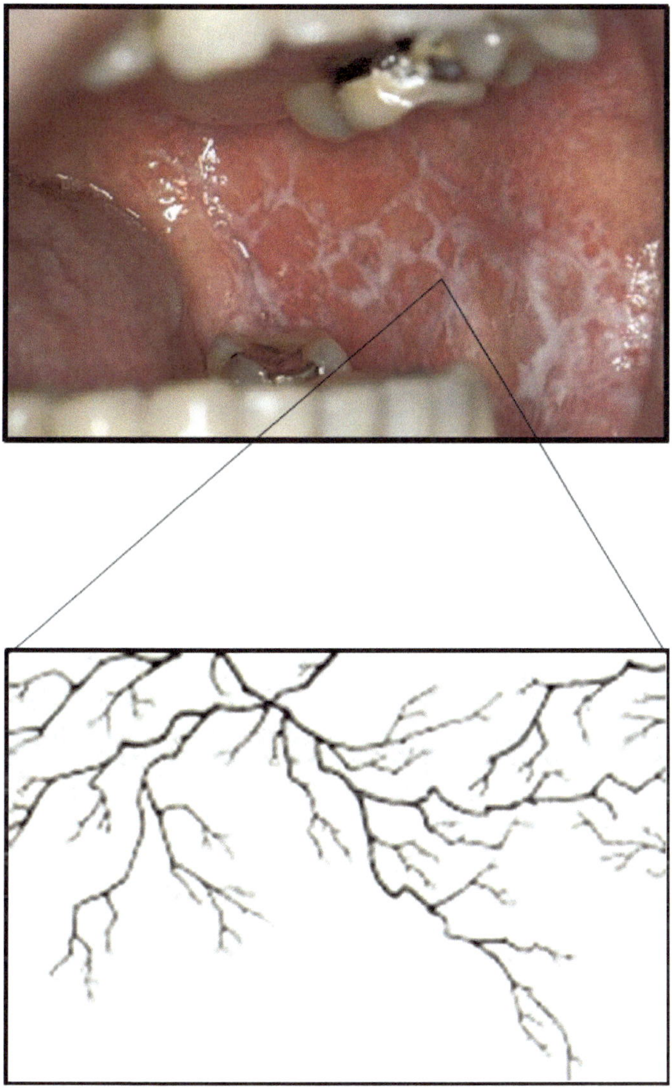

Ślebioda Z, Drożdżyńska J, Karpińska A, Krzyżaniak A, Kasperczak M, Tomoń N, Wiśniewska P, Wyganowska ML. Oral Lichen Planus: Clinical Presentation, Demographic Characteristics, and Risk Factors in a Retrospective Study of 186 Polish Patients. Journal of Clinical Medicine. 2024; 13(23):7363. https://doi.org/10.3390/jcm13237363

WHEN A PATIENT WITH SCARLET FEVER DEVELOPS...

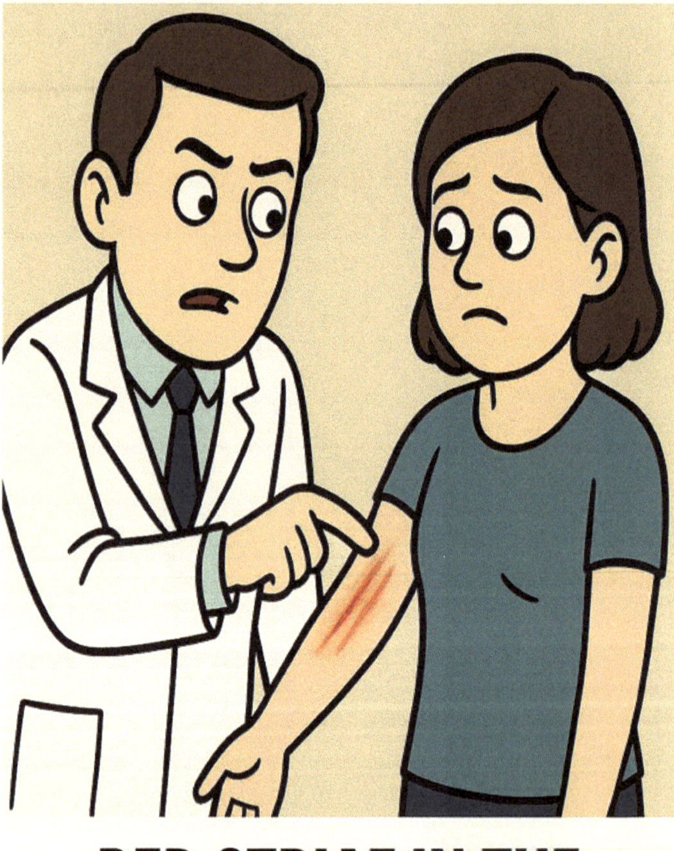

RED STRIAE IN THE FOLD OF THE ARM

Pastia's Lines

- Pastia's lines are a clinical sign characterized by bright red discoloration in skin creases, like those under the arms and in the groin, associated with scarlet fever. They are a pronounced form of the scarlet fever rash in these areas, often appearing before the overall rash develops.
- **Appearance:**
  - ➢ Pastia's lines are typically pink or red and are composed of confluent petechiae (tiny, pinpoint hemorrhages).
- **Location:**
  - ➢ They are found in skin creases, such as the antecubital fossa (the bend of the elbow), axillae (armpits), and groin.
- **Scarlet fever:**
  - ➢ Pastia's lines are a hallmark sign of scarlet fever, a bacterial illness that develops in some individuals with strep throat.
- **Other scarlet fever symptoms:**
  - ➢ Besides Pastia's lines, scarlet fever also presents with additional symptoms like fever, sore throat, and a widespread rash.
- **Treatment:**
  - ➢ Scarlet fever is typically treated with antibiotics, such as penicillin, to eliminate the strep infection.

TREATMENT

Category	Details
Seen In	Scarlet fever – caused by Group A Streptococcus infection
Description	Pink/red linear petechiae in skin folds (e.g., antecubital, axillary) that appear before or along with the rash
Diagnosis	Clinical signs (fever, sore throat, rash, strawberry tongue)- Throat swab (rapid strep test/culture)
Primary Treatment	Antibiotics: Penicillin or amoxicillin (first-line)- Macrolides (if penicillin- allergic)
Supportive Care	Antipyretics (e.g., paracetamol)- Hydration- Rest
Follow-Up	Monitor for complications: rheumatic fever, glomerulonephritis

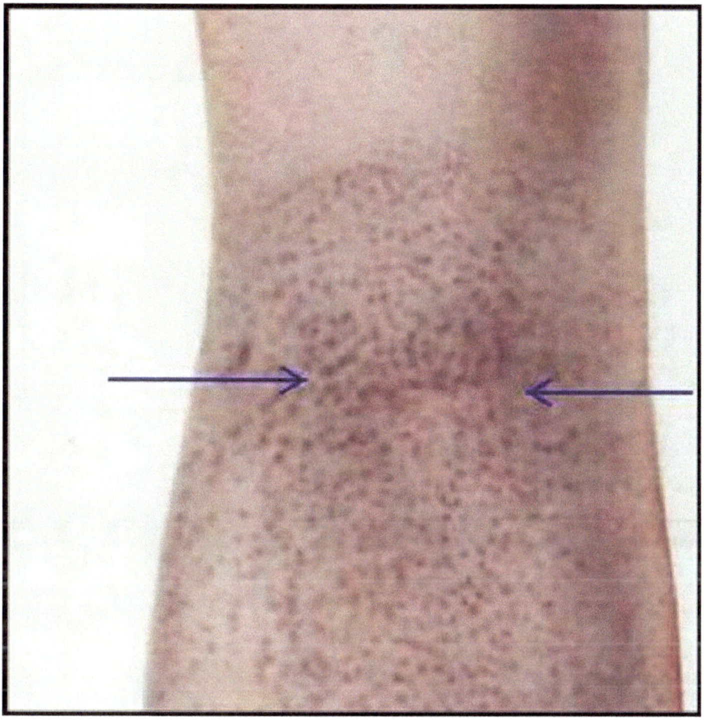

Freiman, Anatoli; Kalia, Sunil; O'Brien, Elizabeth A. (July 2006). "Dermatologic Signs". Journal of 52 Cutaneous Medicine and Surgery. 10 (4): 175–182. doi:10.2310/7750.2006.00042

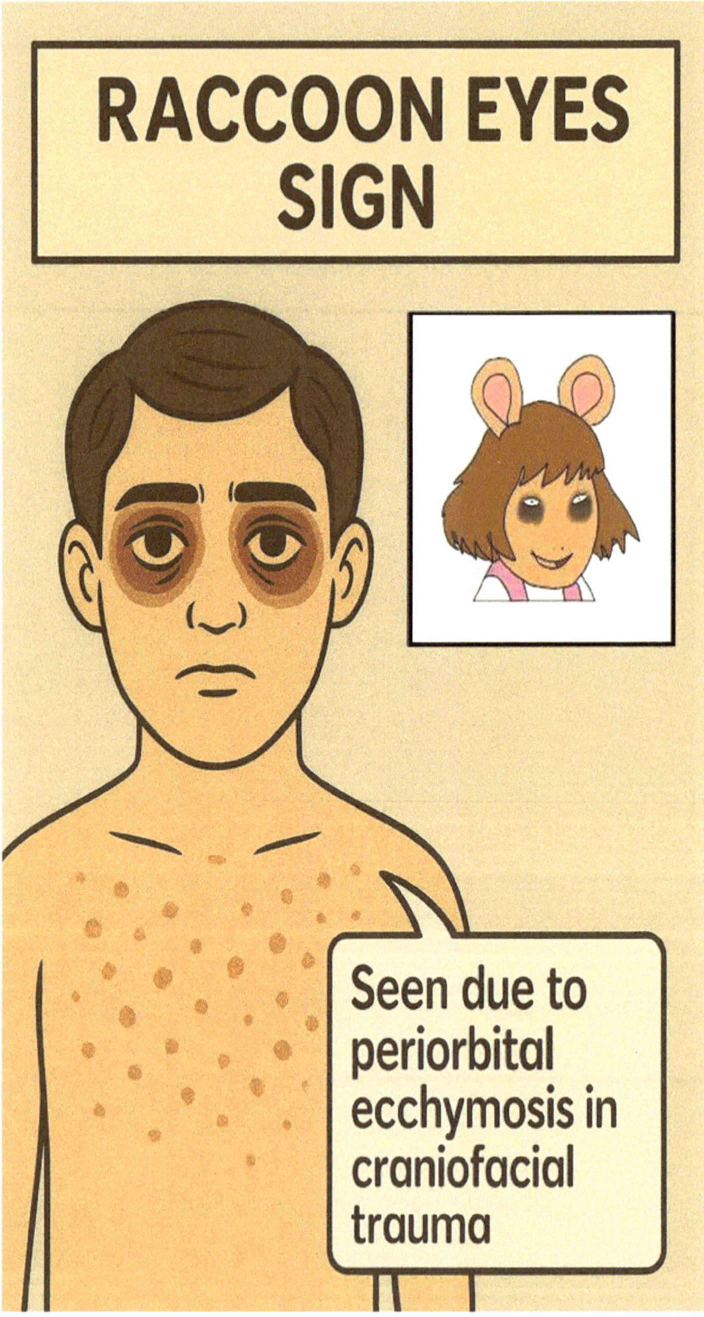
RACCOON EYES SIGN
Seen due to periorbital ecchymosis in craniofacial trauma

RACOON EYES

- Definition: - Involves unilateral or bilateral progressive bruising around the eyes accompanied by swelling.
- This condition is also known as "raccoon eyes" or the "Panda sign."
- Blood accumulation around the eyes is most frequently linked to fractures at the base of the anterior cranial fossa.
- It is not typically seen immediately after the injury and usually manifests 1 to 3 days later.
- If the raccoon sign appears in a trauma patient, it is important to consider the following related injuries and complications that it may indicate:

1. Cerebrospinal fluid (CSF) rhinorrhoea.	6. Insult to the hypothalamic-pituitary axis (HPA) causing endocrinopathies.
2. Injury to the eyeballs.	7. Maxillofacial injuries.
3. Injury to cranial nerves I, II, III, IV, and VI.	8. Cervical spine injury.
4. Intracranial misplacement of the nasogastric or nasotracheal tube.	9. Pneumocephalus.
5. Diffuse axonal injury.	10. Later stage meningitis.

The different causes that can lead to the appearance of the 'Raccoon sign' can be categorized as follows:

1. Traumatic
2. Vascular

3. Infections
4. Immune-mediated
5. Metabolic
6. Malignancies
7. Genetic
8. Iatrogenic

TREATMENT

Category	Details
Seen In	• Basilar skull fracture (anterior cranial fossa) • Orbital trauma • Rarely in neuroblastoma or amyloidosis
Diagnosis	• Clinical sign: bilateral periorbital ecchymosis- Confirm with CT scan of the head- Evaluate for CSF rhinorrhea, Battle's sign, and other skull fracture signs
Primary Treatment	• Stabilization of patient (ABCDE approach) • Neurosurgical consultation if skull fracture present • Monitor for intracranial bleeding or CSF leak
Supportive Care	• Head elevation- Avoid nasal packing or NG tubes if CSF leak suspected • Prophylactic antibiotics if open fracture or CSF leak
Follow-Up	• Neurologic monitoring and follow-up imaging

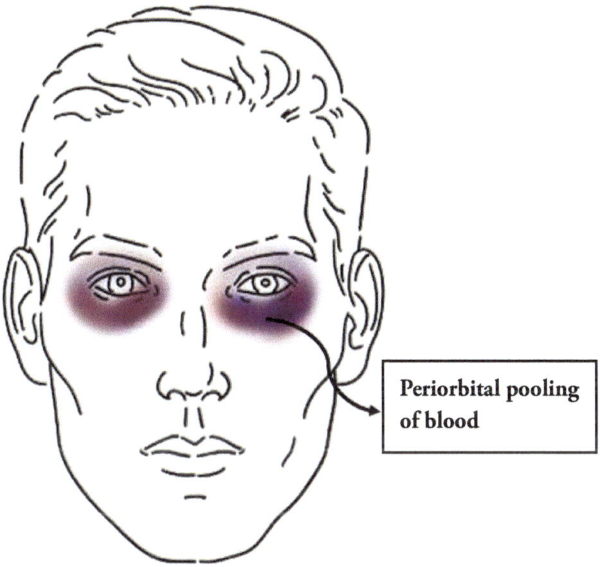
Periorbital pooling
of blood

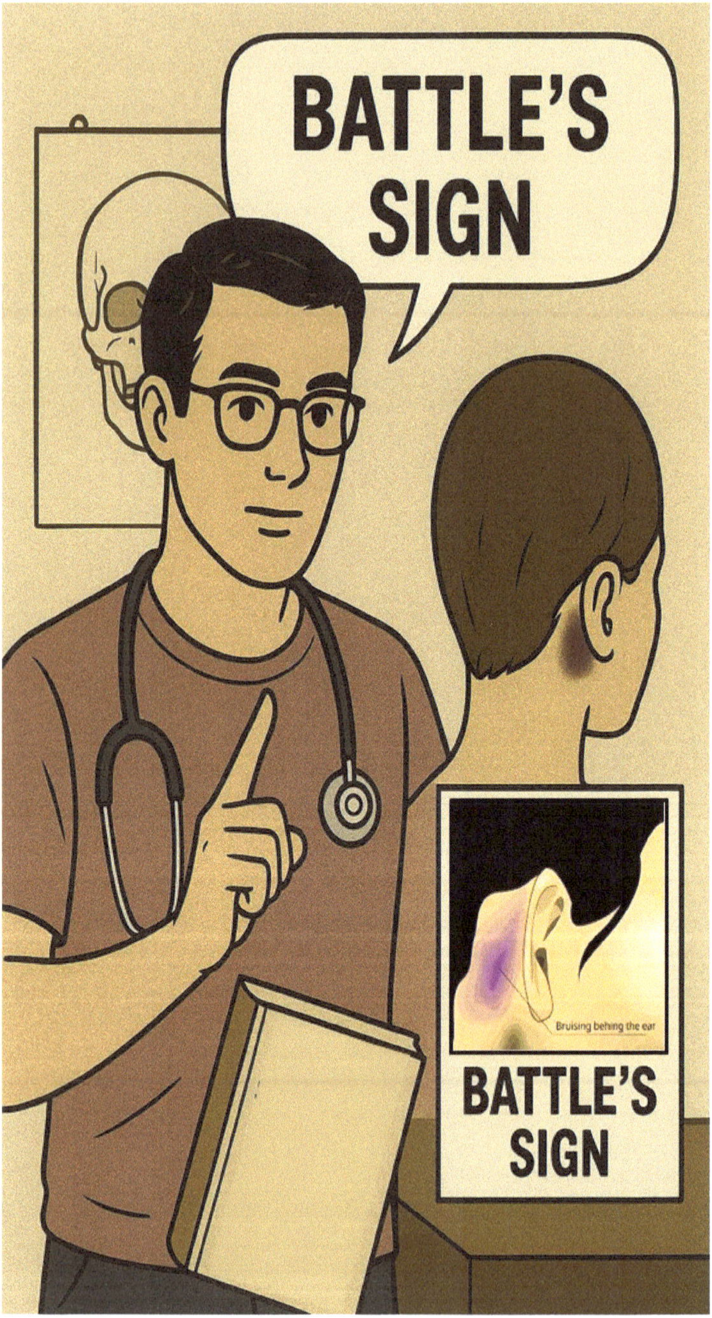
BATTLE'S
SIGN
Bruising behing the ear
BATTLE'S
SIGN

Battle's Sign

- It was **named after** the English surgeon, Dr. William Henry Battle.
- It is a **crescent-shaped bruise** that appears **behind one or both ears** after a person breaks a bone at the base of the skull.
- This type of fracture is known as a **basilar skull fracture**.
- This leads to pooling of blood behind the ear, resulting in the characteristic Battle's sign bruise.
- Battle's sign may not appear right away. It may take a couple of days or more for the bruise to appear after the fracture.
- As a prophylactic measure, anyone who may have suffered a head injury should seek emergency medical care, even in the absence of a bruise.

TREATMENT

Stage	Key Interventions
	• Stabilize patient: Ensure airway, breathing, and circulation (ABCs) • **Neurological assessment:** Monitor consciousness and deficits
Immediate Management	• Pain management: Use analgesics • Prevent secondary injury: Immobilize cervical spine if trauma suspected • Craniotomy: To relieve pressure or repair skull fractures

Surgical Intervention	• Endoscopic repair: Used for cerebrospinal fluid (CSF) leaks • Surgery is considered for brain injury, persistent CSF leak, or infection risk • Physical therapy: For motor recovery • Speech therapy: If communication is affected
Long-term Management	• Regular follow-up: To detect delayed issues like meningitis or ongoing CSF leaks

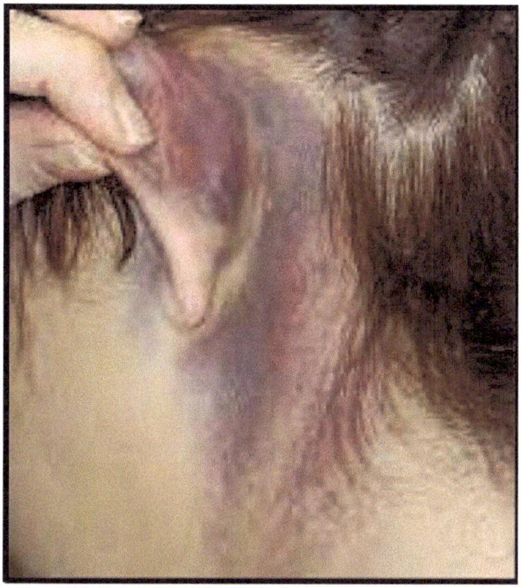

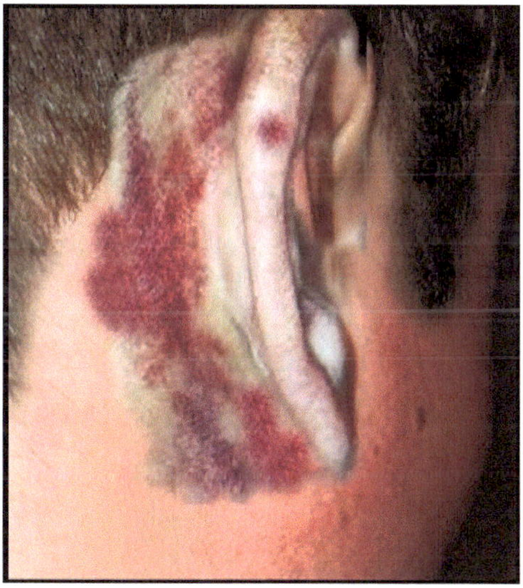

1] https://upload.wikimedia.org/wikipedia/commons/d/d1/Battle_sign_hariadhi.svg. 2] Simon LV, Newton EJ. Basilar Skull Fractures. [Updated 2023 Aug 8]. In: StatPearls [Internet]. Treasure Island (FL): StatPearls Publishing; 2025 Jan-. [Figure, Basilar Skull Fracture, Battle's Sign...] Available from: https://www.ncbi.nlm.nih.gov/sites/books/NBK470175/figure/article-18164.image.f1/

SECTION II

ORAL & ORO-DENTAL SIGNS

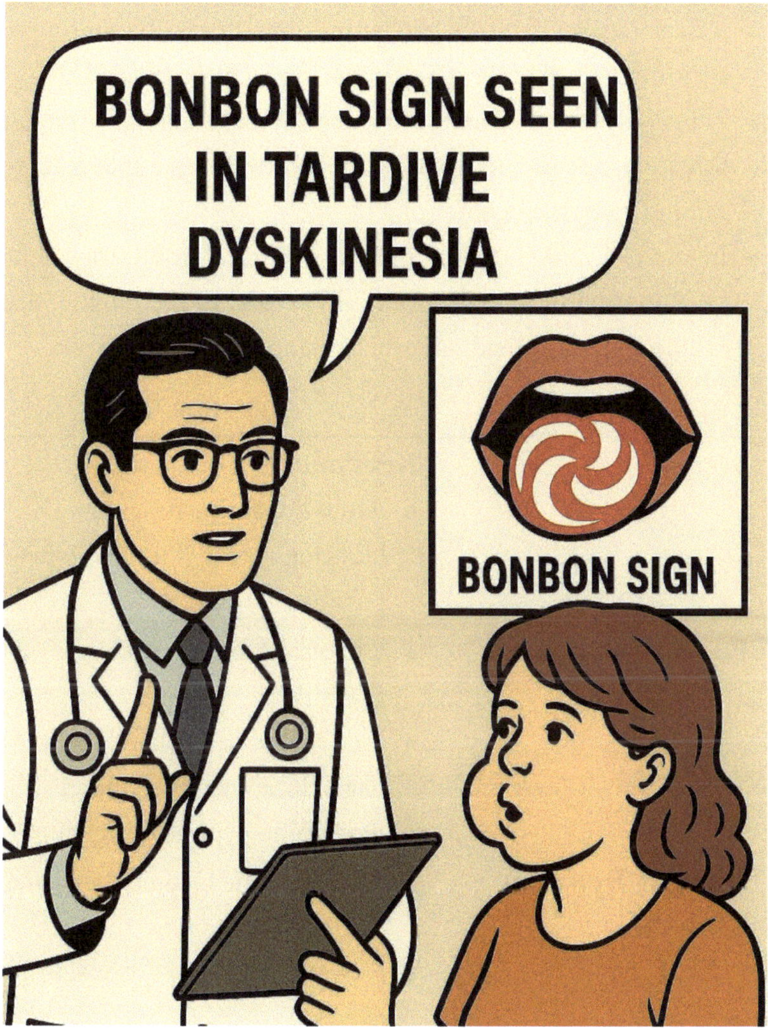
BONBON SIGN SEEN IN TARDIVE DYSKINESIA
BONBON SIGN

Bonbon Sign

- The "bonbon sign" is a clinical sign that helps identify a specific type of movement disorder called Tardive Dyskinesia (TD).
- It is characterized by the patient pressing the tip of their tongue against the cheek as if they were tasting a piece of candy.
- This sign, along with others like the "fly-catching sign" (tongue thrusting out of the mouth) and subtle tongue movements, can indicate the presence of TD.
- In essence, the bonbon sign is a clinical indicator of an involuntary movement, specifically related to the tongue, that can be seen in individuals experiencing tardive dyskinesia.

TREATMENT

Aspect	Key Points
Prevention	• Avoid dopamine receptor-blocking agents (DRBAs) when possible • Use only if no alternatives available • Prefer atypical antipsychotics (e.g., clozapine, quetiapine)
First-line Treatment	• Dopamine-depleting agents: • Tetrabenazine Deutetrabenazine Valbenazine • Newer agents have fewer side effects

Second-line Agents	• Amantadine, clonazepam, ginkgo biloba, zolpidem • Anticholinergics (trihexyphenidyl, benztropine): may help dystonia/ parkinsonism but can worsen TD and cognition
Other Options	• Botulinum toxin: effective for focal (e.g., oromandibular) dystonia
Advanced Treatment	• Deep brain stimulation for severe, treatment- resistant TD

Tardive dyskinesia

- Protrusion and rolling the tongue
- Sucking and smacking movements of lips
- Chewing motion
- Facial dyskinesia
- Involuntary movements of the body and extremities

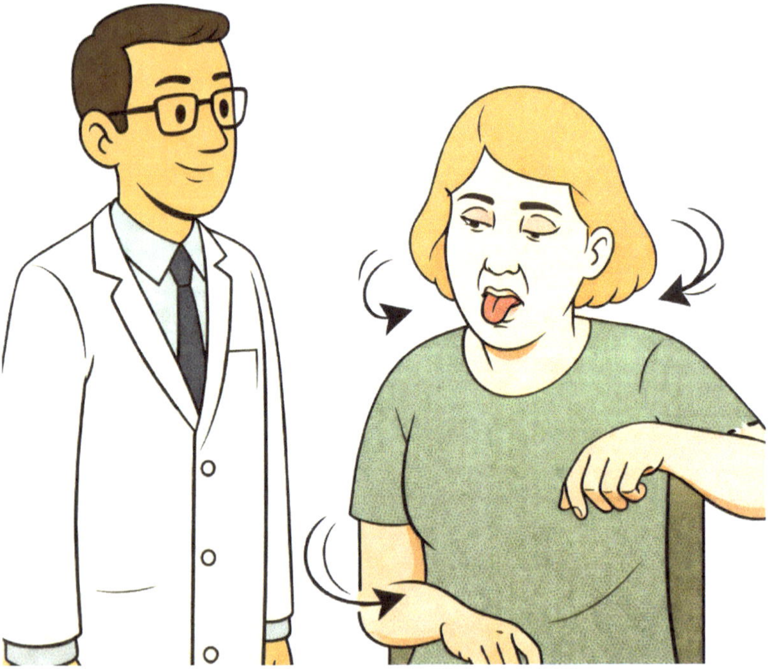

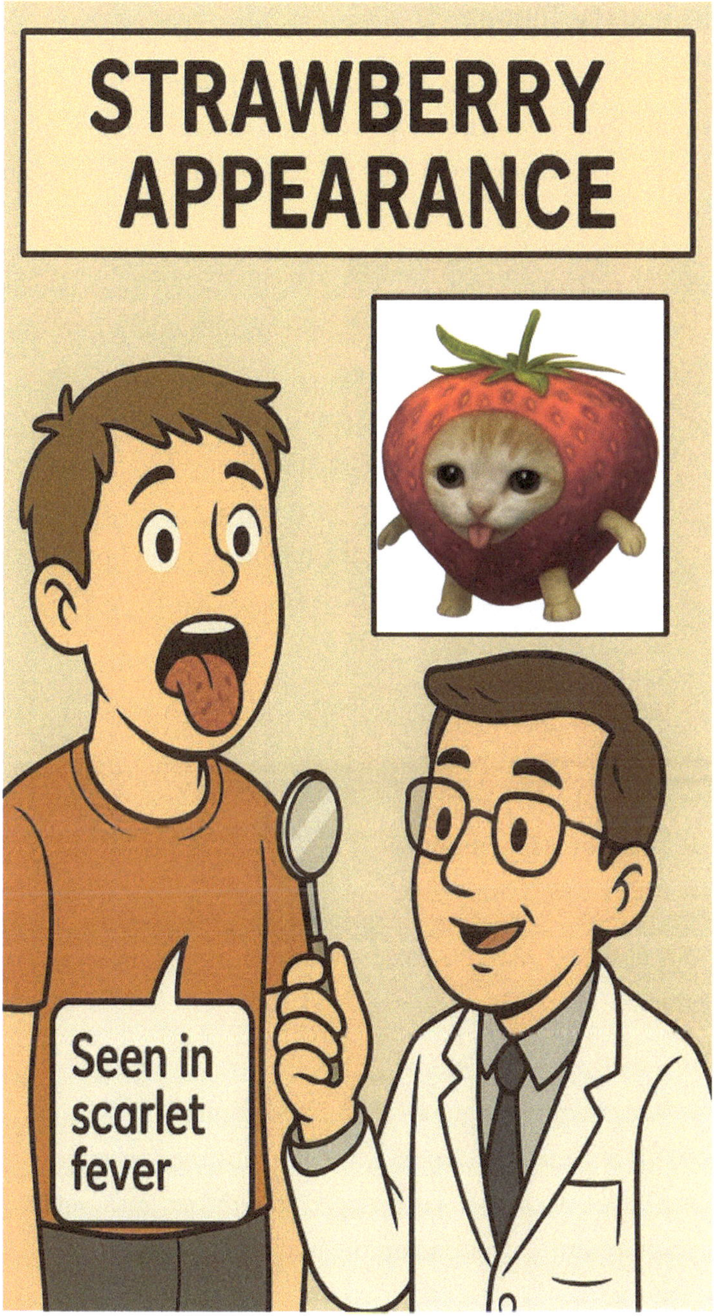
STRAWBERRY APPEARANCE
Seen in scarlet fever

Strawberry Tongue

Strawberry tongue, also known as raspberry tongue, is a condition characterized by a red, bumpy tongue with enlarged taste buds, resembling a strawberry. It's not a disease itself, but a symptom of various underlying conditions.

- **What is it?**
  - ➢ Strawberry tongue is an enanthem, meaning a rash on the inside of the mouth.
  - ➢ It's caused by inflammation and swelling of the fungiform papillae (small, mushroom-shaped bumps) on the tongue.
  - ➢ The papillae may initially be covered by a white coating, which then sheds, leaving the tongue red and bumpy.
  - ➢ While it can be a striking symptom, it's often a sign of a treatable condition.

- **What causes it?**
  - ➢ Scarlet fever
  - ➢ Kawasaki disease
  - ➢ Vitamin B12 deficiency
  - ➢ Other conditions

It can also be linked to toxic shock syndrome and some food allergies.

- **What are the symptoms?**
  - ➢ Red, bumpy tongue with enlarged papillae.
  - ➢ The tongue may appear white initially, then turn red.
  - ➢ May be accompanied by fever, sore throat, rash, and other symptoms depending on the underlying cause.

TREATMENT

Treatment Type	Purpose	Examples/Details
Antibiotics	Treat bacterial infections	Used for scarlet fever, toxic shock syndrome; improvement in a few days
Antihistamines	Reduce allergic reactions	Helps decrease swelling and redness
IV Immunoglobulin (IVIG)	Boost immune response in Kawasaki disease	Given to children; contains human antibodies
Vitamin Supplements	Correct nutritional deficiencies	For B12 or folate deficiency; may include diet changes (e.g., tuna, spinach, beets)

Strawberry tongue

Raspberry tongue

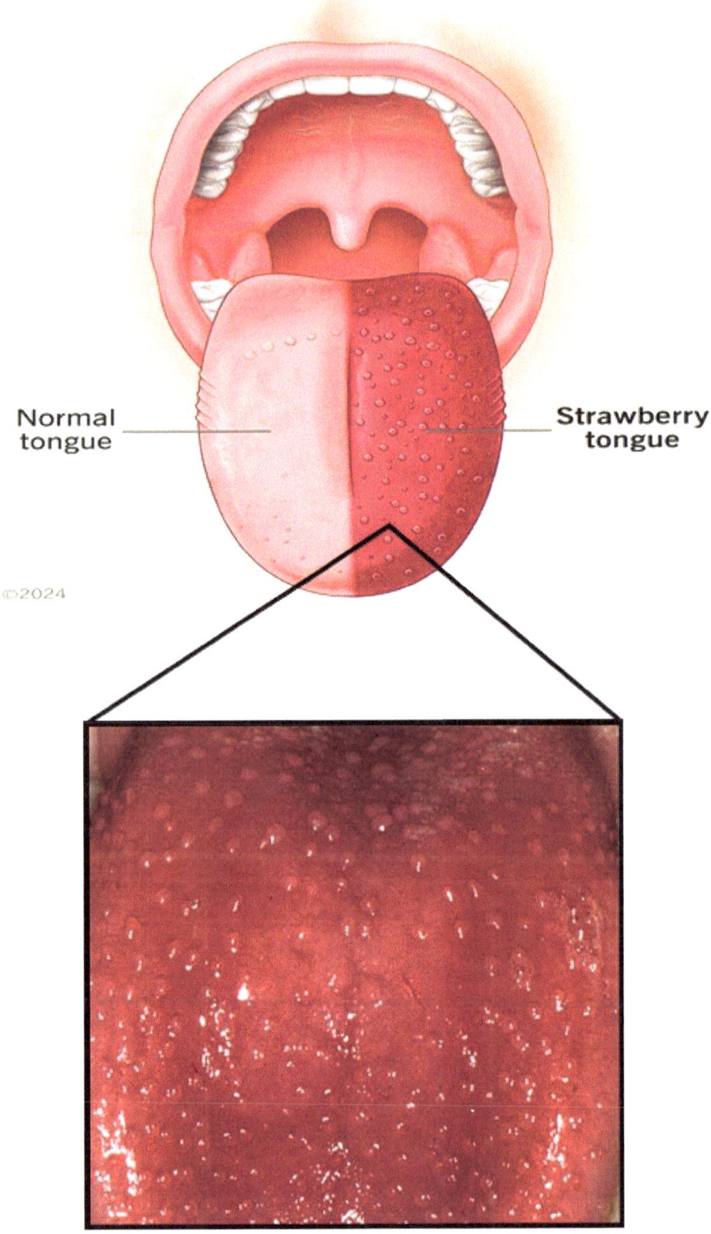

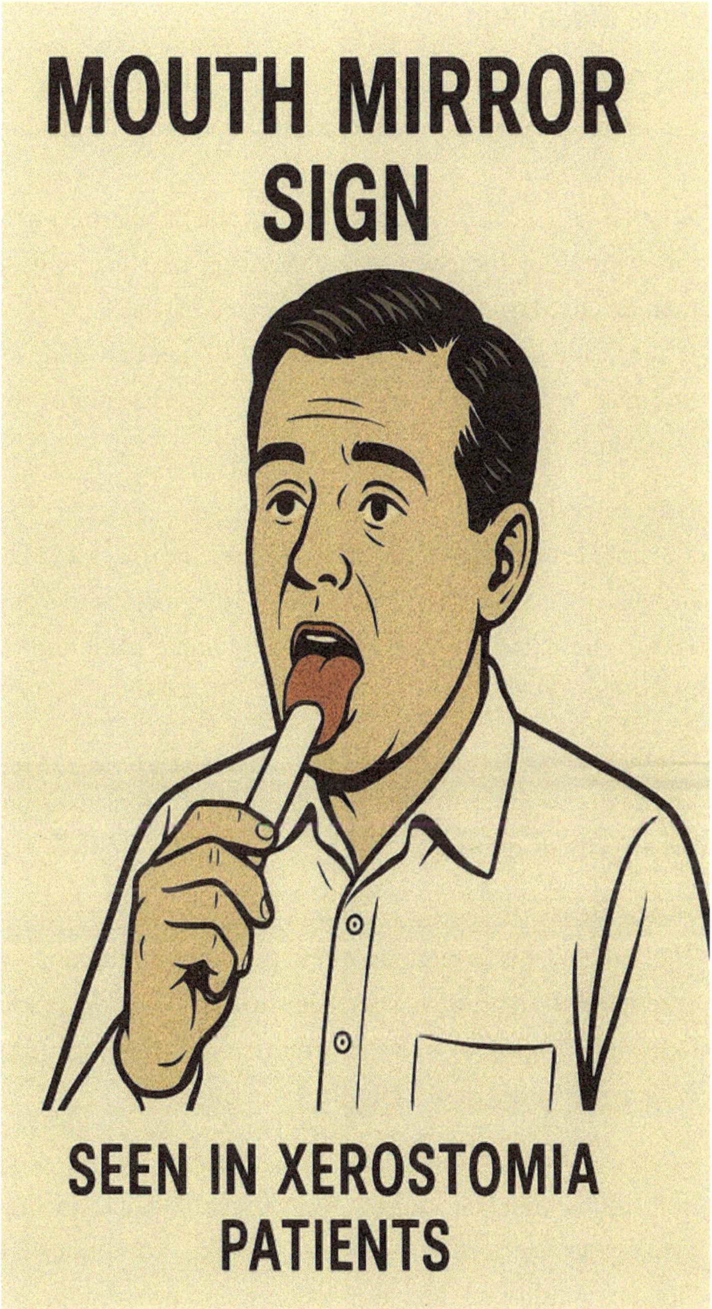
MOUTH MIRROR SIGN
SEEN IN XEROSTOMIA PATIENTS

Tongue Blade Sign

- The "tongue blade sign" (also known as Mouth Mirror Sign) is a simple clinical test used to assess the severity of xerostomia (dry mouth).
- When a tongue blade is pressed against the buccal mucosa (the inner lining of the cheek) for a duration of 10 seconds and then taken away, it should drop off immediately.
- If the blade sticks to the tissue, or is difficult to remove, it indicates reduced salivary flow and suggests more severe xerostomia.

- **How it works:**
  The tongue blade sign relies on the fact that normal saliva keeps the oral tissues moist and lubricated. In xerostomia, reduced salivary flow leads to dryness and the tongue blade can stick to the tissues.

- **Grading Severity:**
  The degree to which the blade sticks can help clinicians estimate the severity of xerostomia.

- **Other Signs:**
  The "tongue blade sign" is often used in conjunction with other clinical signs, such as the "lipstick sign" (lipstick sticking to the front teeth), to assess xerostomia, while investigating the underlying causes of dry mouth.

- **Causes of Xerostomia:**
  Xerostomia can be caused by various factors, including medication side effects, certain medical conditions (like Sjögren's syndrome), radiation therapy, and dehydration.

TREATMENT

Aspect	Key Points
Treat Cause	Stop or adjust causative meds/ drugs if possible
Medication Adjustments	Prefer liquids over tablets, avoid sublingual forms, reschedule doses to reduce night dryness
Symptom Relief	Saliva substitutes- Sugarless fluids- Xylitol gum- Petroleum jelly on lips/dentures
Humidification	Use room or CPAP humidifier at night
Stimulate Saliva	Cevimeline 30 mg TID (less cardiac effect)- Pilocarpine 5 mg TID (more side effects)
Oral Care	Brush, floss, fluoride rinse/gel- Calcium phosphate toothpaste- Avoid sugar near bedtime
Dental Prevention	Fluoride trays at night- Varnish 2–4×/year- Frequent plaque removal visits
Diet Advice	Avoid sugary, acidic, dry, spicy, hot/cold foods

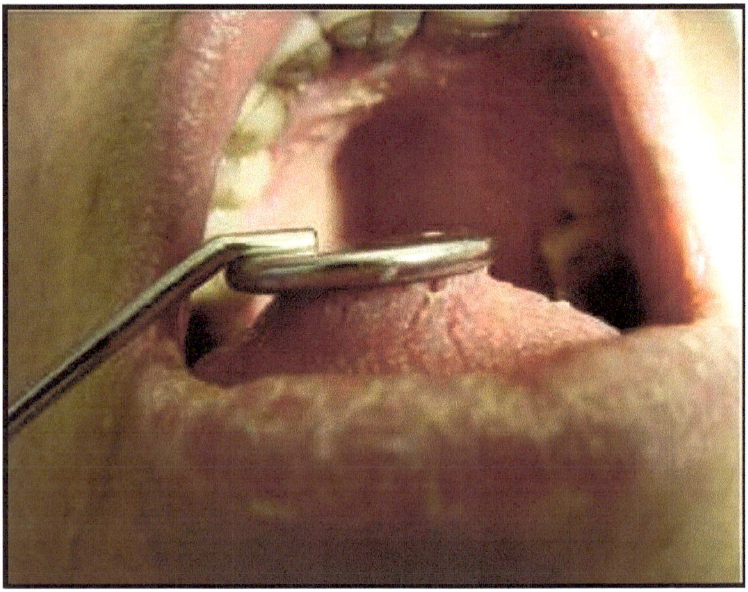

Clinical assessment of oral dryness: development of a scoring system related to salivary flow and mucosal wetness Osailan, S.M. et al. Oral Surgery, Oral Medicine, Oral Pathology and Oral Radiology, Volume 114, Issue 5, 597 - 603

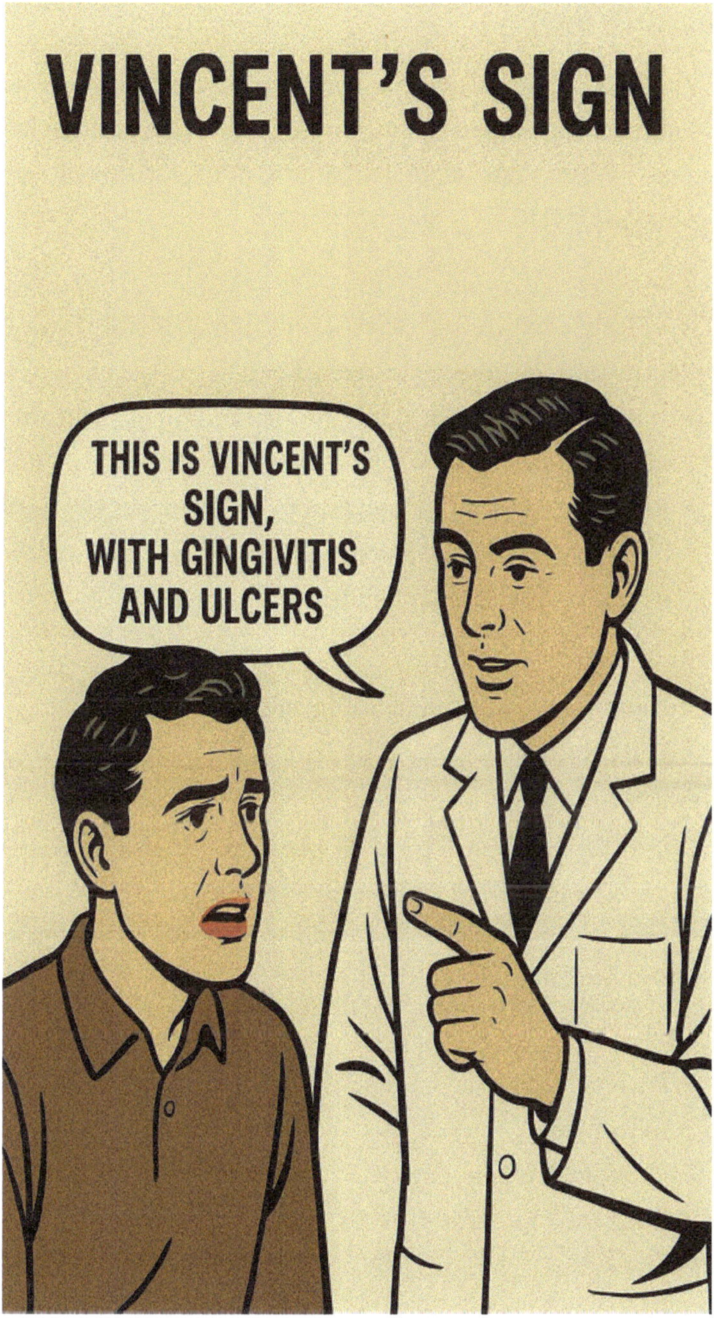
VINCENT'S SIGN
THIS IS VINCENT'S SIGN, WITH GINGIVITIS AND ULCERS

Vincent's Sign

- Vincent's sign, related to dental medicine, pertains to a condition recognized as Vincent's angina, which is also referred to as Vincent's disease, trench mouth, or necrotizing ulcerative gingivitis (NUG).
- **What it is:**
  - ➢ Vincent's angina is a bacterial infection, primarily caused by a fusiform bacillus and a spirochete.
  - ➢ It typically affects the gums, tonsils, and other tissues in the mouth.
  - ➢ The condition is characterized by pain, inflammation, bleeding, and ulceration of the gums, often with a yellowish or grayish pseudo membrane.
- **Symptoms:**
  - ➢ Painful, swollen, and bleeding gums.
  - ➢ Bad breath (halitosis).
  - ➢ Fever.
  - ➢ Swollen lymph nodes in the neck and throat.
  - ➢ Difficulty chewing and swallowing.
  - ➢ Oral ulcers, which may extend to the soft palate, tongue, and buccal mucosa.
- **Causes:**
  - ➢ Bacterial infection, primarily from fusiform bacilli and spirochetes.
  - ➢ Poor oral hygiene.
  - ➢ Weakened immune system.
  - ➢ Stress.

- Nutritional deficiencies.

- **Diagnosis:**
  - Based on clinical symptoms and examination of the mouth.
  - Microscopic examination of scrapings from the lesions may be performed to identify the bacteria.

TREATMENT

Step	Details
1. Oral Hygiene	Prescribe and demonstrate proper oral care and hygiene techniques
2. Antibiotics	If fever, severe gum pain, or bleeding are present – prescribe antibiotics (especially penicillin)
3. Pain Management	Apply topical lidocaine to the gums for relief from pain and swelling
4. Oral Rinses	- Use hydrogen peroxide to rinse the mouth and clear damaged tissue- Saltwater rinses multiple times daily for soothing
5. Dietary Advice	Avoid hot and spicy foods to avoid irritation
6. Professional Cleaning	Once pain and tenderness subside, perform dental cleaning to remove plaque and promote healing

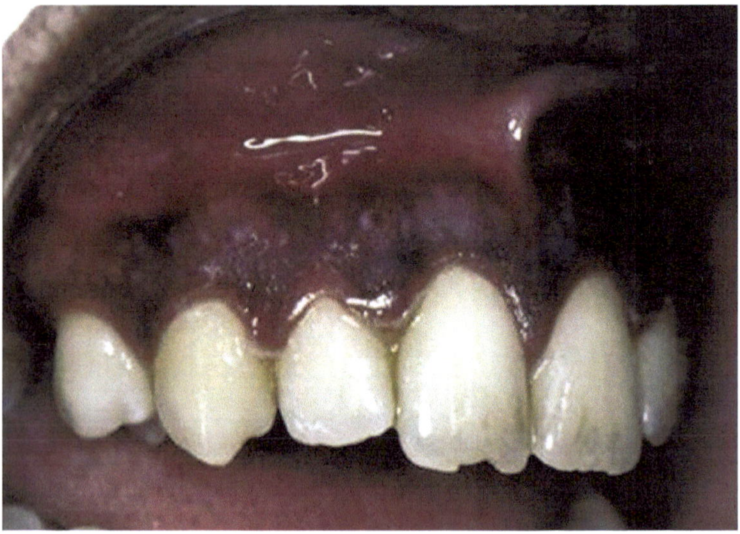

Bhattacharyya S*. Vincent's Angina. Inter Ped Dent Open Acc J 7(4)- 2022. IPDOAJ. MS.ID.000268. DOI: 73 10.32474/IPDOAJ.2022.07.000268

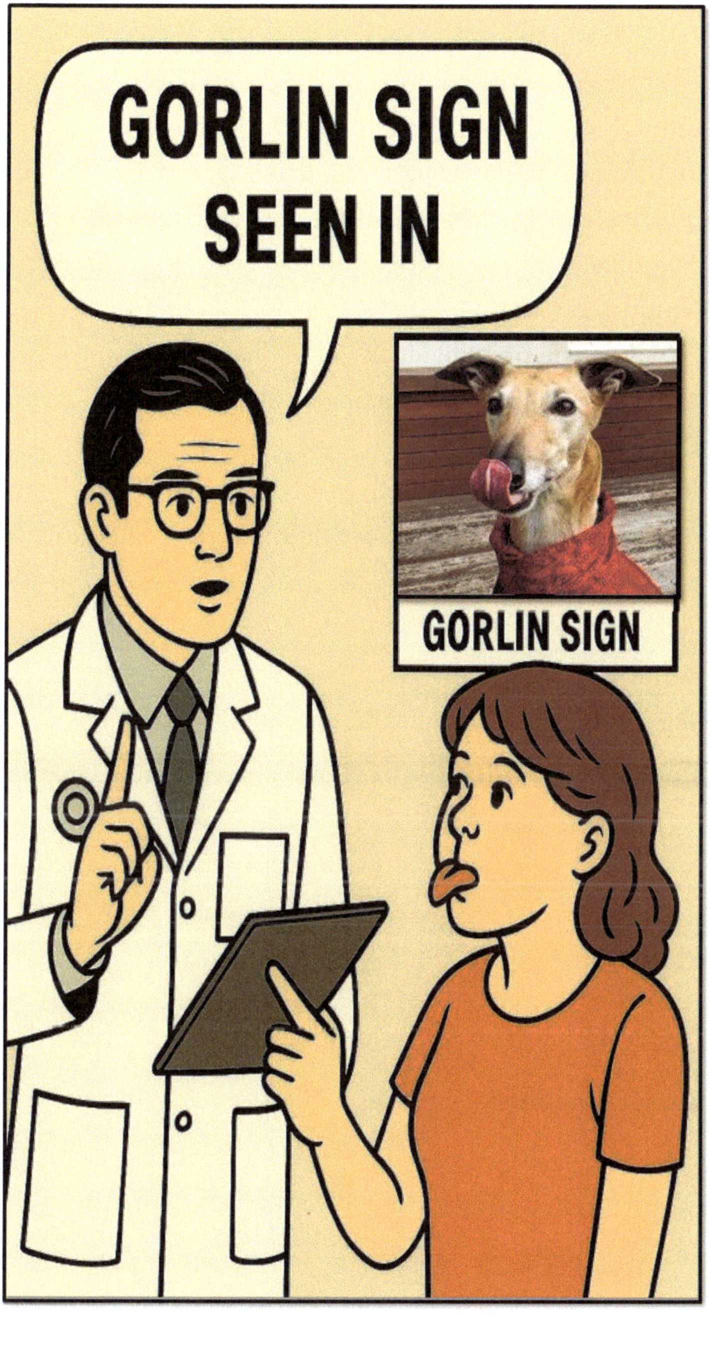
GORLIN SIGN
SEEN IN
GORLIN SIGN

Gorlins Sign

- **First described by** pathologist Robert J. Gorlin, in twentieth century medical literature.
- **Definition:-** It is a medical term that indicates the ability of an individual to touch the tip of the nose with the tongue.
- Approximately ten percent of the general population can perform this act.
- Fifty percent of individuals with Ehlers–Danlos syndrome, a hereditary disorder affecting connective tissue, have this characteristic.
- It should not be confused with Gorlin syndrome, another major hereditary medical condition named after the same pathologist.

TREATMENT

Focus Area	Management Strategies
Joint Hypermobility	• Physical therapy to strengthen muscles • Joint protection and bracing when required
Skin Fragility	• Gentle skin care • Avoid trauma or excessive pressure
Pain Management	• Analgesics • Physical therapy • Sometimes low-dose antidepressants or gabapentin

Cardiac Monitoring	• Regular check-ups for mitral valve prolapse or aortic root dilation (in some EDS types)
Genetic Counselling	• Especially for inherited connective tissue disorders like EDS

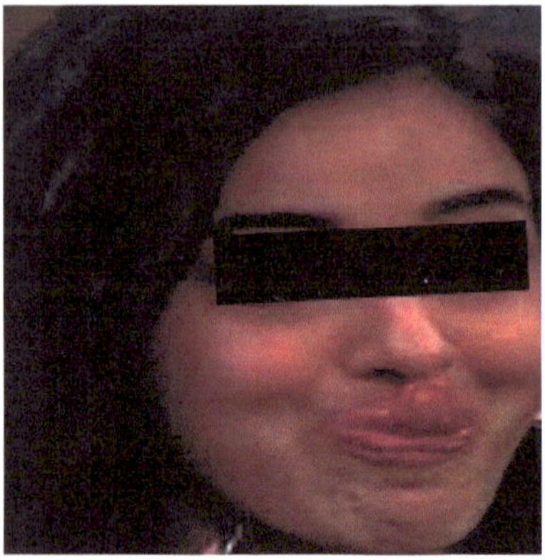

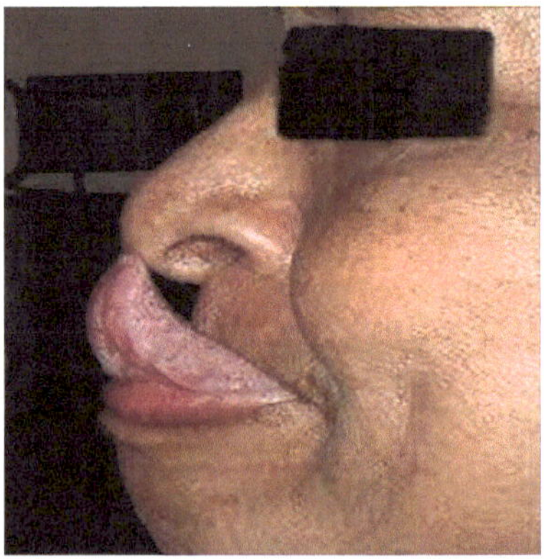

Kassam, Karim; Cascarini, Luke (6 March 2014). "Gorlin's sign". BMJ. 348: g1786. doi:10.1136/bmj.g1786. ISSN 1756- 1833

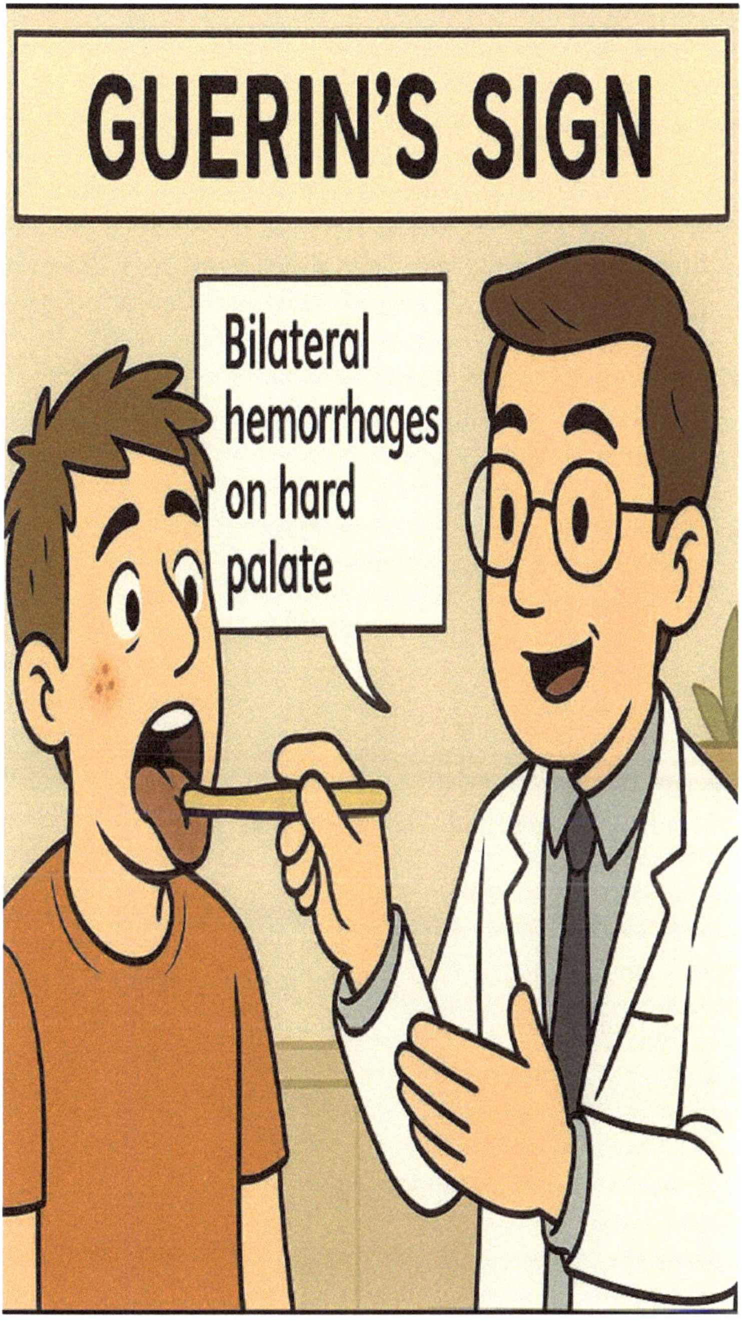
GUERIN'S SIGN
Bilateral hemorrhages on hard palate

Guerrin Sign

- Sir Alphonse François Marie Guérin (1816-1895) described Guerin's sign in Le Fort I Fracture.
- It is bruising and ecchymosis on the palate in the region of the Greater palatine arteries resulting from a force of injury directed low on the maxillary alveolar rim in a downward direction.

- **Location:**
  - ➢ Bruising and swelling in the palate, specifically around the greater palatine foramen.

- **Cause:**
  - ➢ Typically caused by blunt force trauma to the face, often in the context of assaults, road traffic accidents, or falls.

- **Associated injuries:**
  - ➢ Le Fort I fracture (a horizontal fracture of the maxilla), fractures of the palatine bone and pterygoid process of the sphenoid bone, and sometimes a mid- palatal split.

- **Clinical significance:**
  - ➢ Guerin's sign is a valuable clinical clue in diagnosing midfacial fractures and guiding further diagnostic imaging and treatment.

- **Diagnosis:**
  - ➢ Identified through clinical examination, and CT scans can confirm the extent and pattern of fractures.

- **Management:**
  - ➢ Treatment involves addressing the fracture and associated injuries, infection control, and managing swelling and pain.

TREATMENT

Category	Management Approach
Initial Care	• Stabilize ABCs (Airway, Breathing, Circulation) • Control bleeding- Assess for head/spine injury
Diagnosis	• CT scan (maxillofacial) for detailed fracture mapping • Clinical exam for midface mobility
Definitive Treatment	• Open reduction and internal fixation (ORIF) • Surgical stabilization of the maxilla
Follow-up	• Dental and ENT evaluation • Monitor for malocclusion, sinus issues, or infection

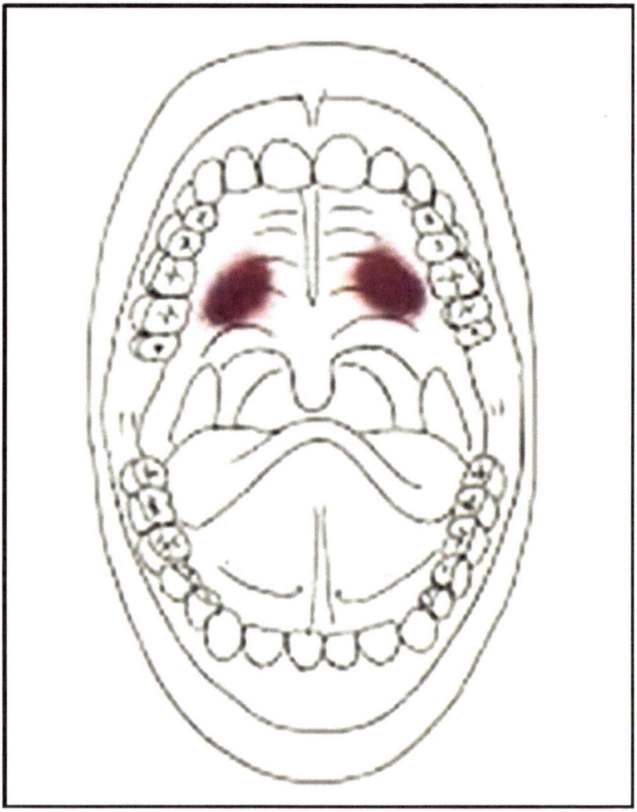

IOSR Journal of Dental and Medical Sciences (IOSR-JDMS) e-ISSN: 2279-0853, p-ISSN: 2279-0861.Volume 22, Issue 11 Ser.2 (November. 2023), PP 58-65

WHEN YOU SEE TINY WHITE SPOTS ON THE BUCCAL MUCOSA...

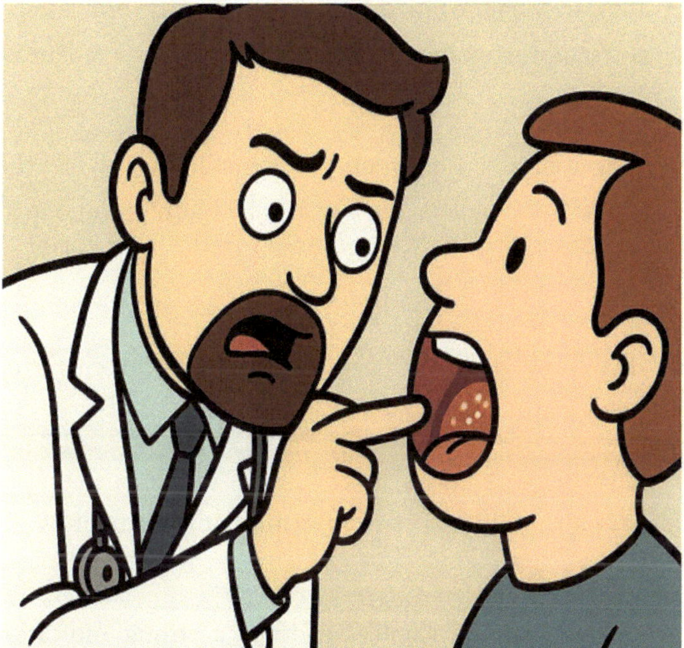

BETTER CANCEL THAT PLAYDATE. IT'S MEASLES

Koplik's Spots

Koplik's spots are tiny, white or bluish-white lesions with a red outline that form on the mucous membrane of the cheeks, usually in proximity to the molars. They are a key diagnostic sign for measles.

- **Appearance:**
  - ➢ 'Ihey are small, white or bluish-white spots (often described as resembling grains of sand) surrounded by a red area.
- **Location:**
  - ➢ They typically appear on the inner lining of the cheeks, opposite the molars, but can also be found in other parts of the mouth.
- **Timing:**
  - ➢ They usually appear 2-3 days before the characteristic measles rash.
- **Duration:**
  - ➢ They are usually short-lived, lasting only a day or two.
- **Pathognomonic:**
  - ➢ The presence of Koplik's spots is a strong indication of measles, helping differentiate it from other viral illnesses.

TREATMENT

Aspect	Management
Supportive Care	• Rest, fluids, antipyretics (e.g. paracetamol). • Monitor for complications.
Vitamin A	• Supplementation reduces morbidity and mortality in children.
Isolation	• Prevent spread (measles is highly contagious).
Prevention	• MMR vaccine (measles, mumps, rubella).

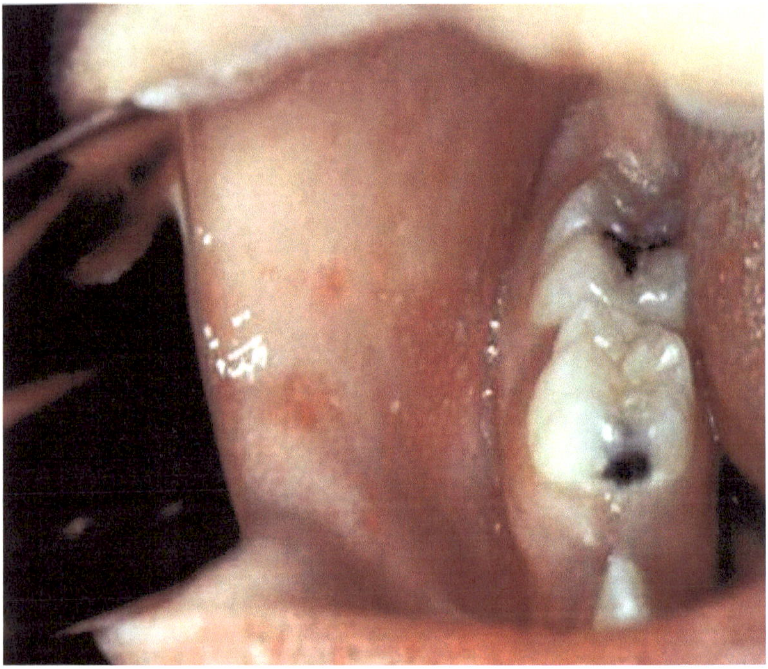

http://phil.cdc.gov/PHIL_Images/20040908/4f54ee8f0e5f49f58aaa30c1bc
6413ba/6111_lores.jpg

SECTION III

CARDIOVASCULAR & HAEMATOLOGICAL SIGNS

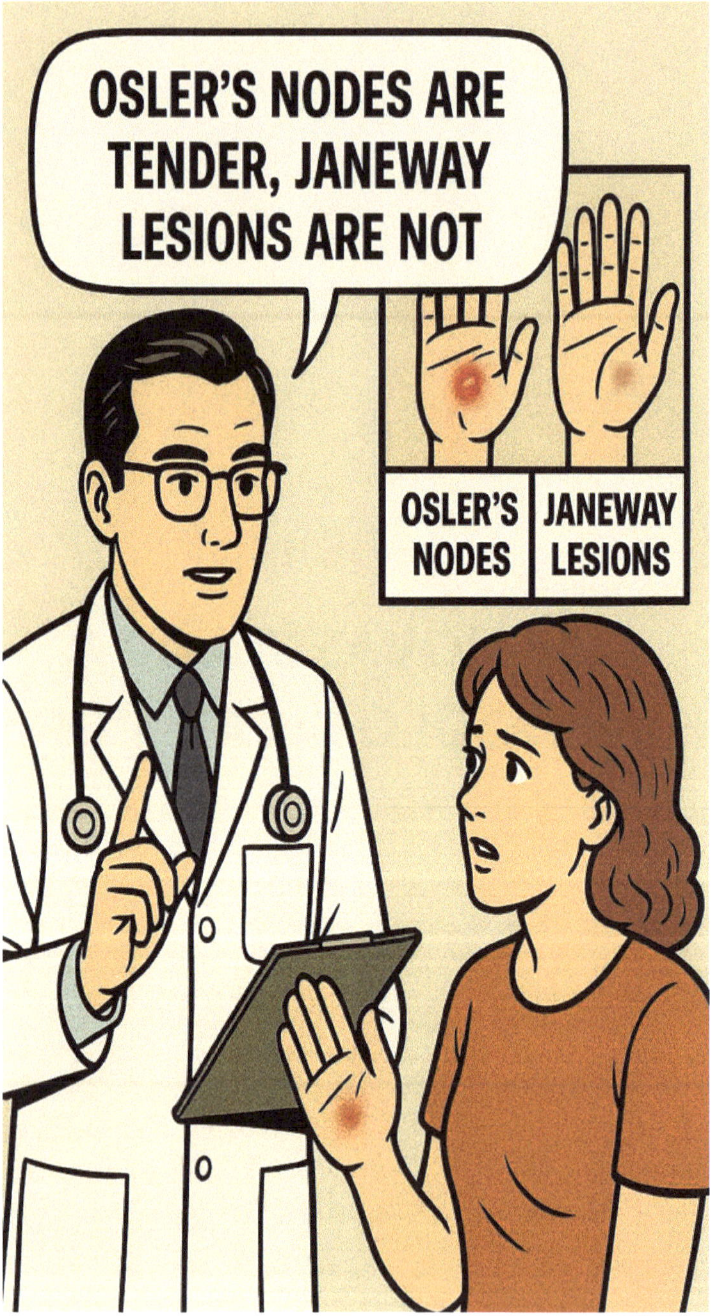
OSLER'S NODES ARE TENDER, JANEWAY LESIONS ARE NOT
OSLER'S NODES
JANEWAY LESIONS

Osler Nodes and Janeway Lesions

- Dr. William Osler initially identified Osler nodes in 1893, while Dr. Edward Janeway described Janeway lesions in 1899.
- Both Osler nodes and Janeway lesions are skin symptoms associated with endocarditis, a condition usually caused by a bacterial or fungal infection of the heart's endocardium.

Feature	Osler Nodes	Janeway Lesions
Tenderness	Tender	Non-tender
Appearance	Purplish-pink nodules	Erythematous or hemorrhagic macules
Size	1–1.5 mm	Variable
Location	Finger/toe tips, thenar/ hypothen ar	Palms and soles
Pathology	Immune complex-mediated vasculitis	Septic emboli causing microabscesses
Duration	Hours to days	Days to weeks
Histology	Neutrophilic infiltration, vasculitis	Bacterial colonies in dermis

TREATMENT

Feature	Osler Nodes	Janeway Lesions
Seen In	Infective endocarditis	Infective endocarditis
Cause	Immune complex deposition (Type III hypersensitivity)	Septic micro emboli (infectious material)
Appearance	Painful, red/purple nodules	Painless, flat red macules
Location	Finger/toe pads, thenar/ hypothenar eminences	Palms and soles
Associated Symptoms	Fever, murmurs, embolic signs	Fever, murmurs, embolic signs
Diagnosis	- Clinical exam- Blood cultures- Echocardiography	Same as Osler nodes
Primary Treatment	IV antibiotics (e.g., penicillin, vancomycin, gentamicin) for 4–6 weeks	
Supportive Care	Pain relief if needed	Usually none required due to painless nature
Follow-Up	Monitor for complications (e.g., embolism, heart failure)	Same

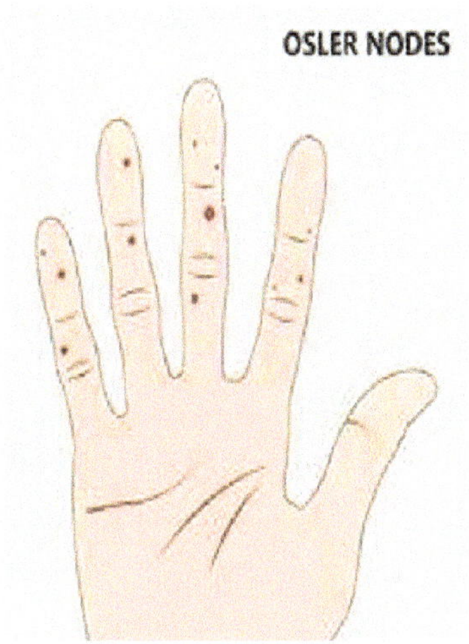
OSLER NODES

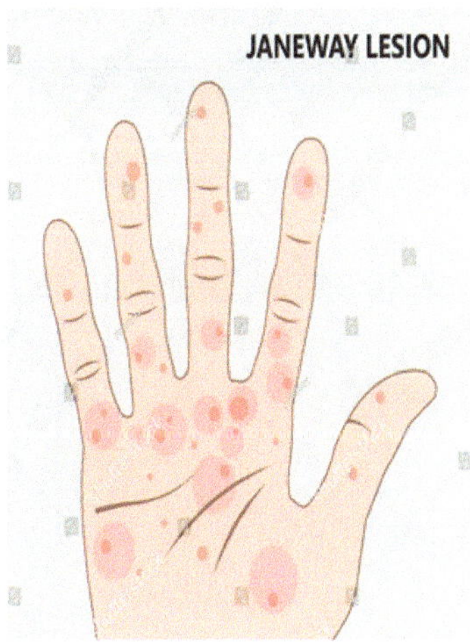
JANEWAY LESION

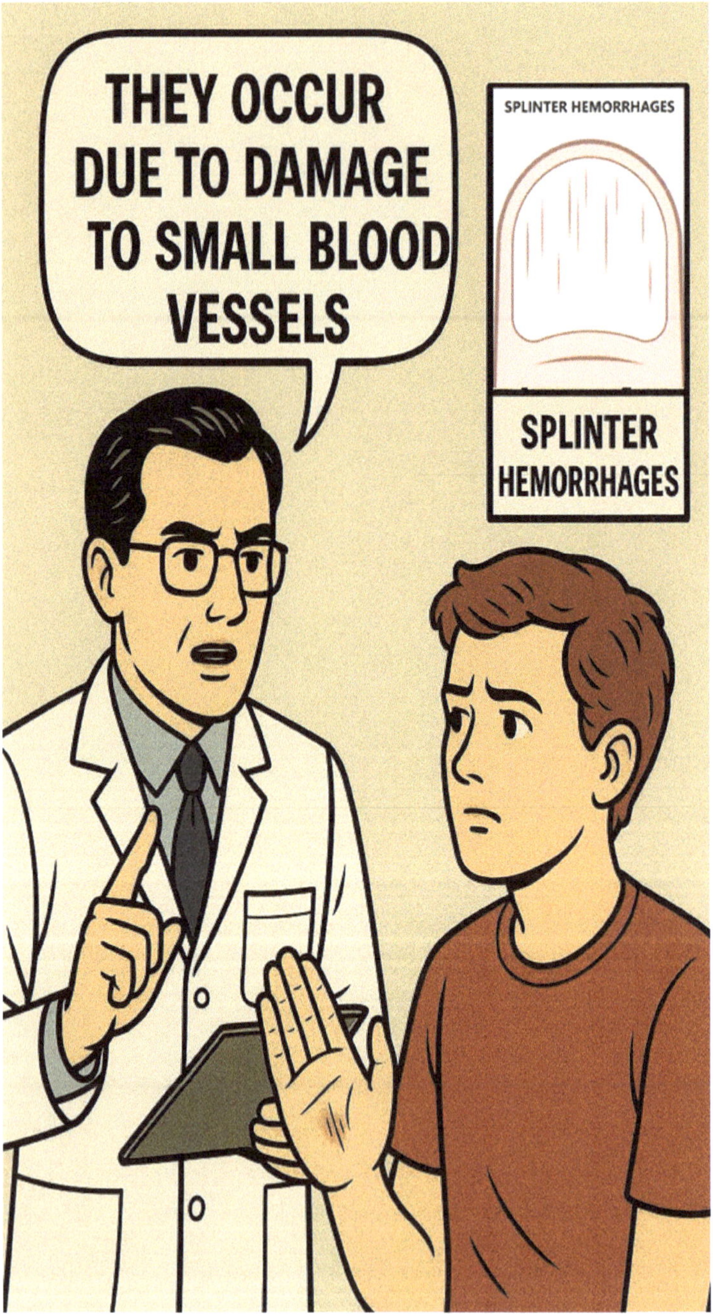
THEY OCCUR DUE TO DAMAGE TO SMALL BLOOD VESSELS
SPLINTER HEMORRHAGES
SPLINTER HEMORRHAGES

Splinter Haemorrhage

Splinter hemorrhages are typically thin, red to reddish- brown streaks that run vertically along the nail, following its growth direction.

- **Causes:**
  1. **Trauma:** Injuries to the nail, such as a finger or toe, can damage the blood vessels and cause splinter hemorrhages.
  2. **Underlying Conditions:** In some cases, they can be a sign of conditions like:
     - Infective Endocarditis: An infection of the heart valves.
     - Vasculitis: Inflammation of blood vessels.
     - Antiphospholipid Syndrome: An autoimmune disorder.
     - Other Systemic Diseases: Lupus, Raynaud's phenomenon, and even trichinosis can also be associated with splinter hemorrhages.

- **Symptoms:**

  Splinter hemorrhages are often painless, but they can be painful if caused by a recent injury.

- **Diagnosis:**

  A doctor can diagnose splinter hemorrhages through a physical examination and may order further tests (like a complete blood count or blood cultures) depending on the suspected cause.

- **Treatment:**

  The treatment focuses on adressing the root cause of the bleeding. For example, if endocarditis is the cause, antibiotics are required.

TREATMENT

Category	Details
Seen In	• Subacute bacterial endocarditis (classic)- Trauma- Vasculitis- Autoimmune diseases (e.g., SLE, RA)
Diagnosis	• Clinical nail examination- Blood cultures if infective endocarditis is suspected- Echocardiography for cardiac evaluation
Primary Treatment	• Depends on the underlying cause:- Infective Endocarditis → IV antibiotics- Autoimmune cause → Immunosuppressive therapy- Trauma → No specific treatment needed
Supportive Care	• Nail care and monitoring; treat any local secondary infection if present
Follow-Up	• Regular monitoring of systemic condition and resolution of hemorrhages

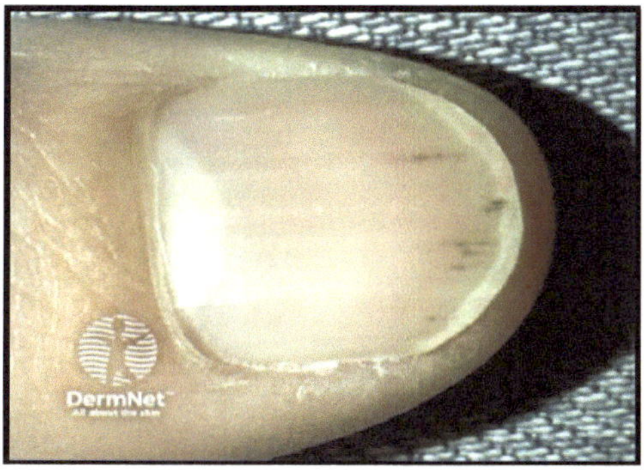

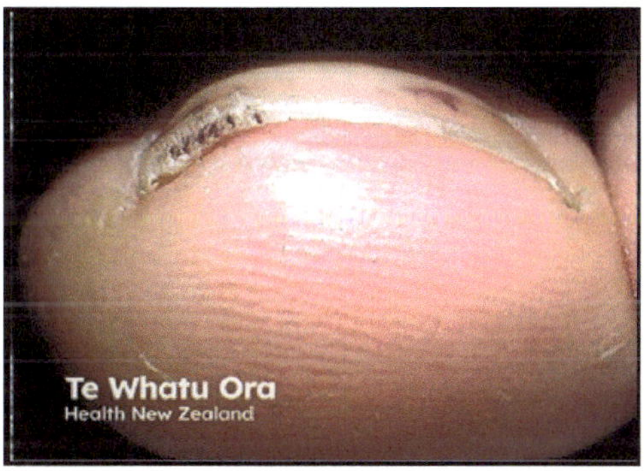

Dr Alice Manley, Core Medical Trainee, Southmead Hospital, North Bristol Trust, United Kingdom. DermNet Editor in Chief: A/Prof. Amanda Oakley, Dermatologist, Hamilton, New Zealand. Copy edited by Gus Mitchell. February 2019. https://dermnetnz.org/

SECTION IV

NEUROLOGICAL & MUSCULOSKELETAL SIGNS

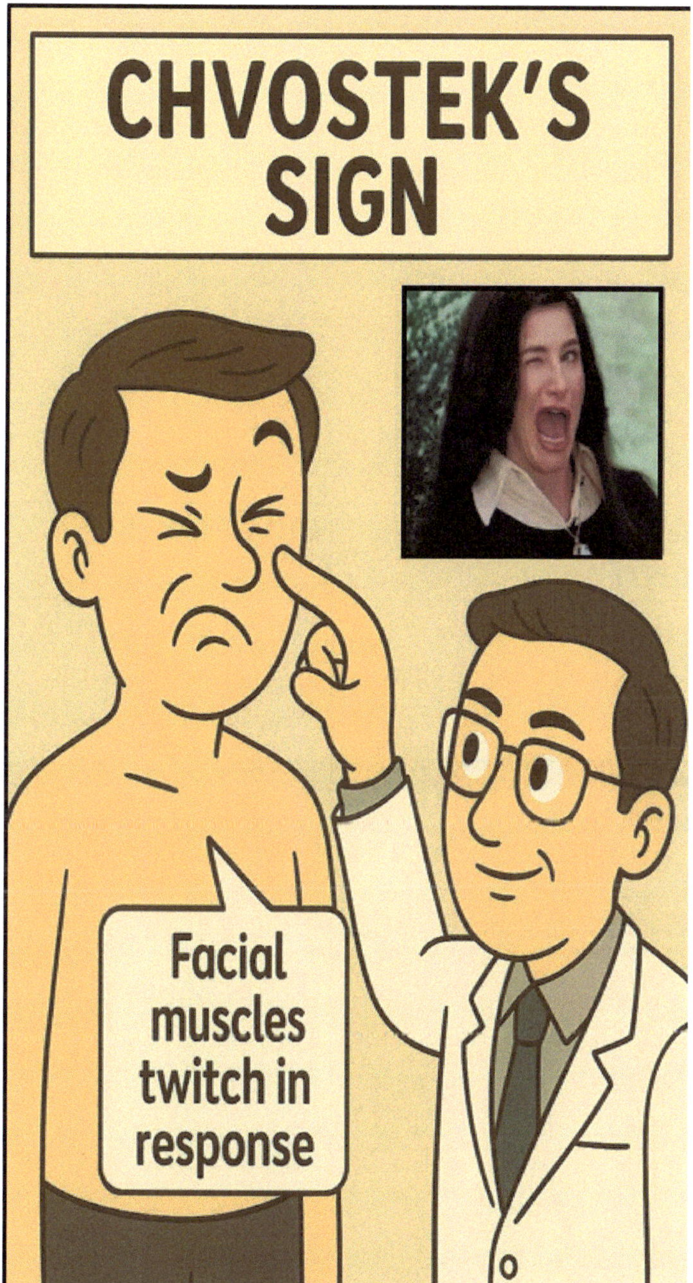
CHVOSTEK'S SIGN
Facial muscles twitch in response

Chvostek Sign

- Given by Frantisek Chvostek.
- It is one of the tetany symptoms associated with hypocalcemia..
- It refers to an abnormal reaction to the stimulation of the facial nerve.
- **May be encountered in:**
  - Respiratory alkalosis like hyperventilation.
  - Rickets.
  - Diphtheria.
  - Measles.

Chvostek phenomenon:- CHVOSTEK I	CHVOSTEK II
• Contracture of facial muscles elicited by tapping on the facial nerve at a specific point which is located ➢ 0.5 to 1 cm lower to the zygomatic ➢ process of the temporal bone ➢ 2cm front to the ear lobe, ➢ on a line with the angle of mandible.	• It can be produced by tapping on different location of the face which is located ➢ On the line joining the zygomatic prominence and corner of mouth, 1/3rd of distance from the zygoma.

TREATMENT

Treatment Component	Details
Calcium Supplementation	• Oral calcium (e.g., calcium carbonate or citrate) to raise serum calcium levels
Vitamin D Supplementation	• Enhances calcium absorption • Given if vitamin D levels are low
Intravenous Calcium	• For severe hypocalcemia or symptoms (e.g., muscle spasms)-Typically calcium gluconate, given in hospital
Treat Underlying Cause	• Depends on the origin (e.g., hypoparathyroidism, vitamin D deficiency, drug-induced) • May include recombinant parathyroid hormone
Monitoring & Follow-up	• Regular checks of calcium levels • Adjust treatment as needed for long-term control

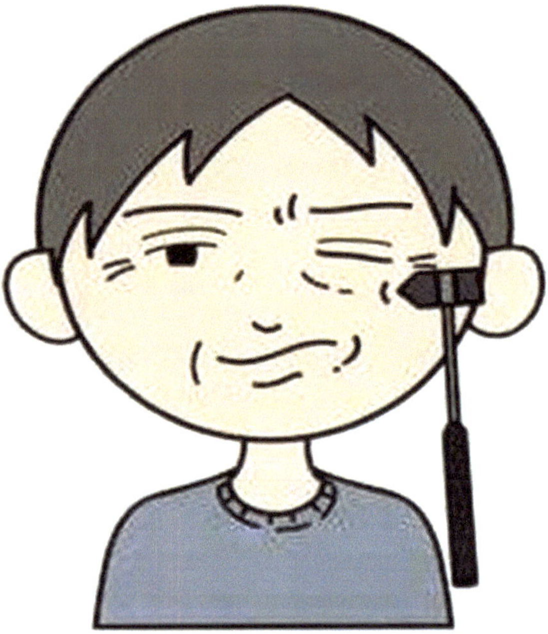

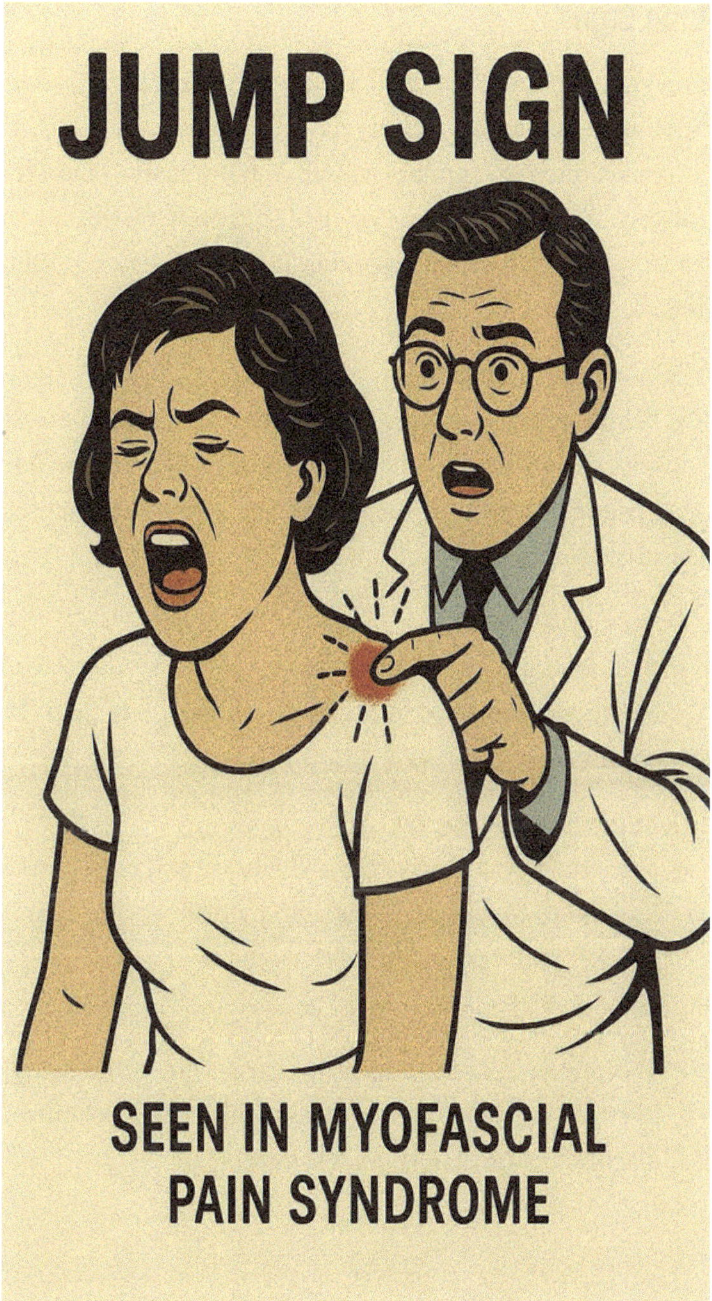
JUMP SIGN
SEEN IN MYOFASCIAL
PAIN SYNDROME

Jump Sign

In myofascial pain syndrome (MPS), a jump sign is a characteristic response to palpation of a myofascial trigger point (TP). It's a noticeable, often involuntary, twitch or movement of the affected muscle or surrounding tissue when a TP is pressed. This response, also called a local twitch response, is a key diagnostic sign for MPS.

- **Palpation and Pressure:**
  - When a myofascial trigger point is palpated, especially with deep pressure, the patient may experience a sudden, involuntary contraction or twitch in the affected muscle or surrounding area.
- **Response to Pressure:**
  - This response can range from a subtle twitch to a more noticeable jump or movement of the body part being examined.
- **Involuntary Movement:**
  - The twitch or jump is often involuntary and not a conscious reaction to the pressure, making it a distinct sign compared to other pain responses.
- **Diagnostic Significance:**
  - The presence of a jump sign, along with other signs like referred pain and taut muscle bands , helps confirm the diagnosis of myofascial pain syndrome.

TREATMENT

Approach	Details
Physical Therapy	• Stretching, ultrasound, TENS, heat/cold therapy.
Trigger Point Therapy	• Manual release, dry needling, or injections.
Occlusal Appliances	• Night guards/splints to reduce bruxism-related stress.
Medications	• NSAIDs, muscle relaxants, low-dose tricyclic antidepressants.
Behavioural Therapy	• Stress reduction, biofeedback, cognitive behavioral therapy (CBT).

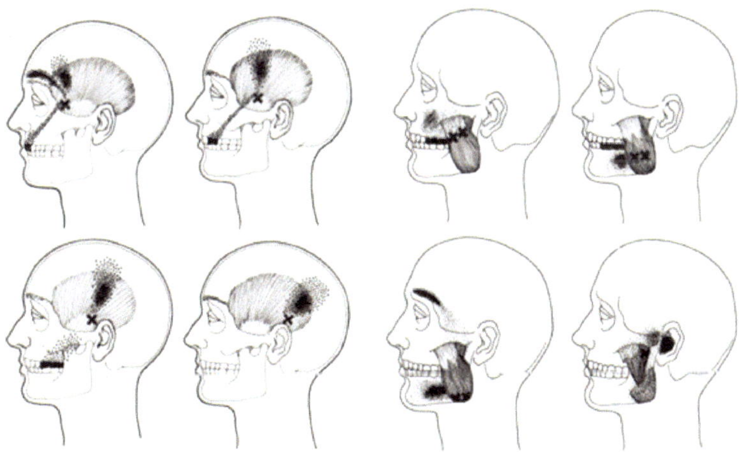

SECTION V

SYSTEMIC & MISCELLANEOUS DIAGNOSTIC SIGNS

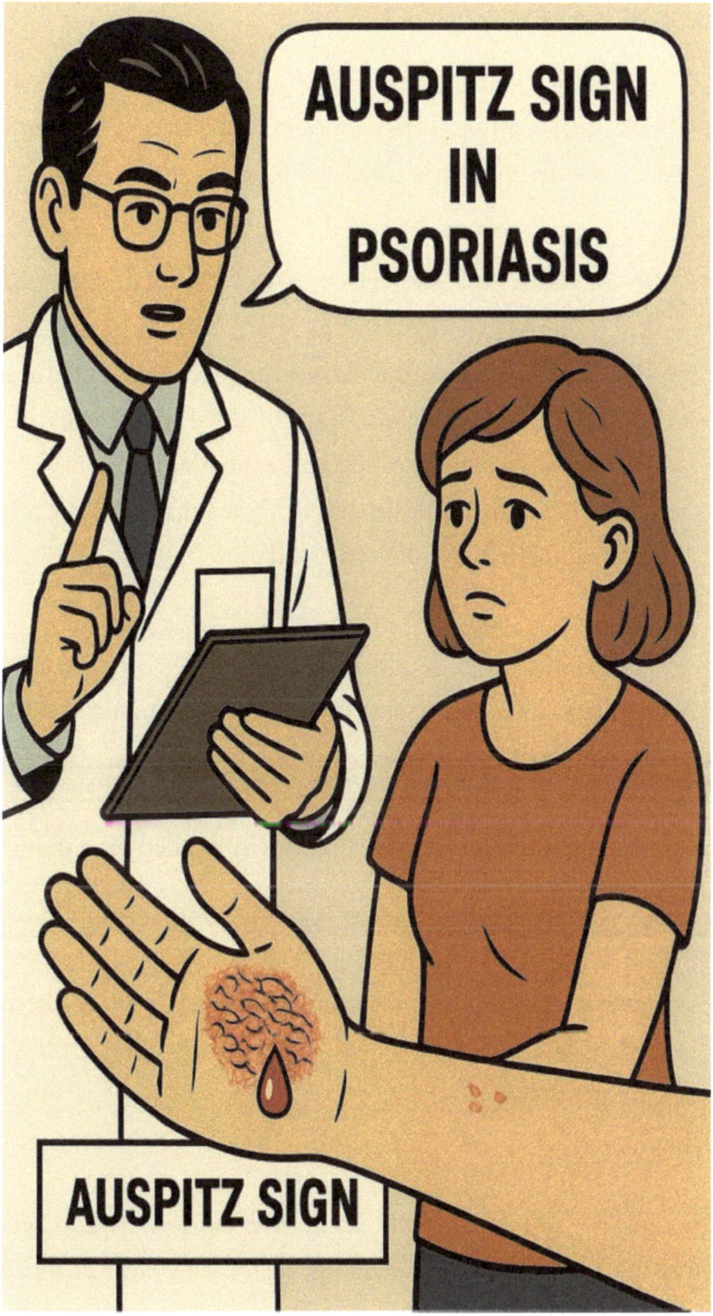
AUSPITZ SIGN
IN
PSORIASIS
AUSPITZ SIGN

Auspitz's Sign

- Described by Sir Heinrich Auspitz (1835-1886)
- The Auspitz sign is a medical sign characterized by pinpoint bleeding when psoriatic scales are scraped off.

- **What it is?**
    - ➢ When you scrape away the scales of a psoriatic plaque, the skin underneath may bleed in small, dot-like patterns.
    - ➢ This occurs because the skin layer (epidermis) is thinned, and the tiny blood vessels (capillaries) at the tips of the dermal papillae are exposed and easily damaged.
    - ➢ The distinctive pinpoint bleeding is caused by rupture of these elongated and dilated capillaries.

- **Why it's important?**
    - ➢ The Auspitz sign is a helpful clinical sign for diagnosing psoriasis, but it's not always present and can also be found in other skin conditions.
    - ➢ Its presence can suggest psoriasis, but further examination and other diagnostic tools are usually needed for a definitive diagnosis.

- **Note:**
    - ➢ Auspitz sign is not a reliable indicator of psoriasis severity and is absent in certain types of psoriasis like pustular and erythrodermic psoriasis.

TREATMENT

Doctors do not specifically treat the Auspitz sign itself. If removing a plaque causes bleeding, they may cover the area and recommend topical agents to prevent infection. However, the most effective approach is to focus on treating the underlying condition responsible for the sign.

Condition	Treatment Options
Psoriasis	• Topical creams and ointments. • Light therapy (phototherapy). • Oral or injectable medications.
Actinic Keratosis	• May go away on its own (can return with sun exposure). • Topical creams or gels to remove spots. • Laser therapy- Light therapy. • Scraping- Cryotherapy (freezing).
Darier's Disease	• Avoid heat and use sunscreen. • Topical steroids or antiseptics to reduce inflammation and bacterial growth. • Oral or topical retinoids.

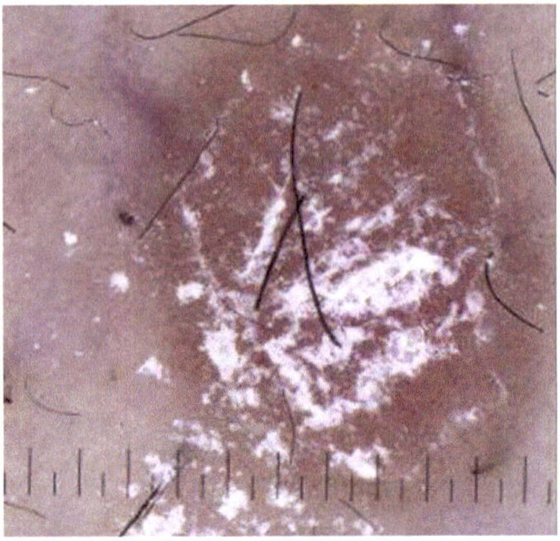

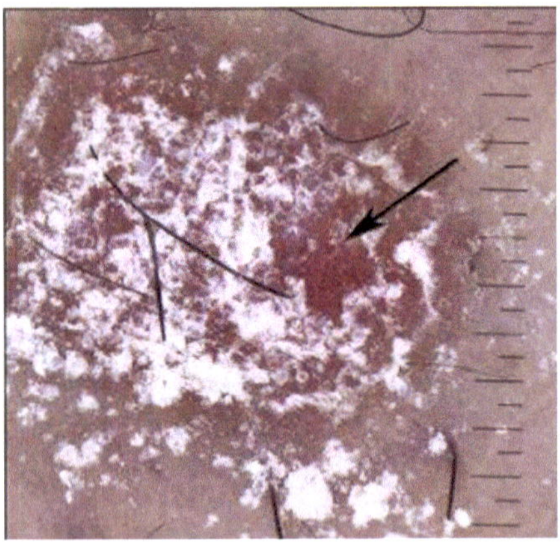

Kaliyadan F. The dermoscopic auspitz sign. Indian Dermatol Online J 2018;9:290-1

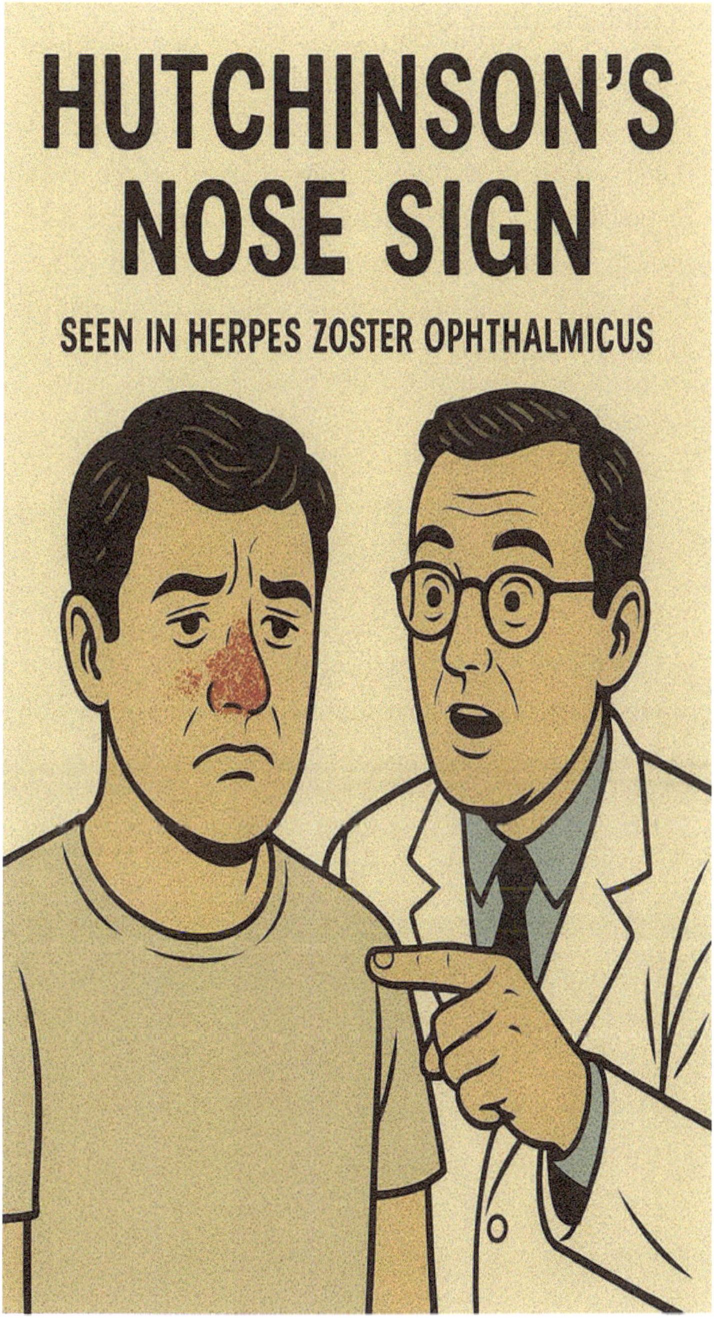
HUTCHINSON'S
NOSE SIGN
SEEN IN HERPES ZOSTER OPHTHALMICUS

Hutchinson's Nose Sign

- Named after Sir Jonathan Hutchinson.
- Describes a rash or blister located on the tip of the nose, which is a characteristic indication of involvement of the nasociliary branch of the ophthalmic division of the trigeminal nerve.
- It's a significant predictor of ocular complications with herpes zoster ophthalmicus (HZO), including uveitis, keratitis, and potentially blindness.

- **Key Points:**
  - **Herpes Zoster Ophthalmicus (HZO):**
    This is a form of shingles affecting the ophthalmic nerve, including the nasociliary branch.
  - **Ocular Complications:**
    Hutchinson's sign raises the risk of serious eye inflammation, such as uveitis and keratitis, and the possibility of vision loss.
  - **Anatomical Significance:**
    The nasociliary branch innervates the tip of the nose, the eye, and parts of the eyelids.
  - **Prognostic Value:**
    Presence of Hutchinson's sign suggests a higher likelihood of developing ocular complications.

TREATMENT

Category	Approach
Urgent Referral	• Immediate referral to an ophthalmologist.
Antiviral Therapy	• Oral antiviral agents (within 72 hrs. of rash onset): • **Acyclovir,** • **Valacyclovir** • **Famciclovir**
Pain Management	• Analgesics, gabapentin/ pregabalin for neuropathic pain.
Eye Care	• Topical corticosteroids or antivirals **under specialist guidance** if eye involvement is confirmed.
Follow-Up	• Monitor for complications such as postherpetic neuralgia, keratitis, or vision changes.

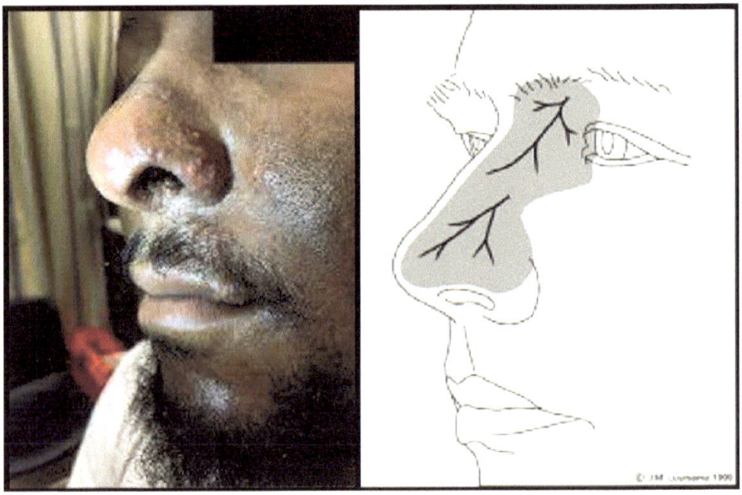

1]Lawrence Lau, MD*, Hannah Mirzakhani, BA^ and Nicholas Governatori, MD DOI: https://doi.org/10.21980/J8N0402] Zaal, M.J.W., Völker-Dieben, H.J. & D'Amaro, J. Prognostic value of Hutchinson's sign in acute herpes zoster ophthalmicus. Graefe's Arch Clin Exp Ophthalmol 241, 187–191 (2003). https://doi.org/10.1007/s00417-002-0609-1

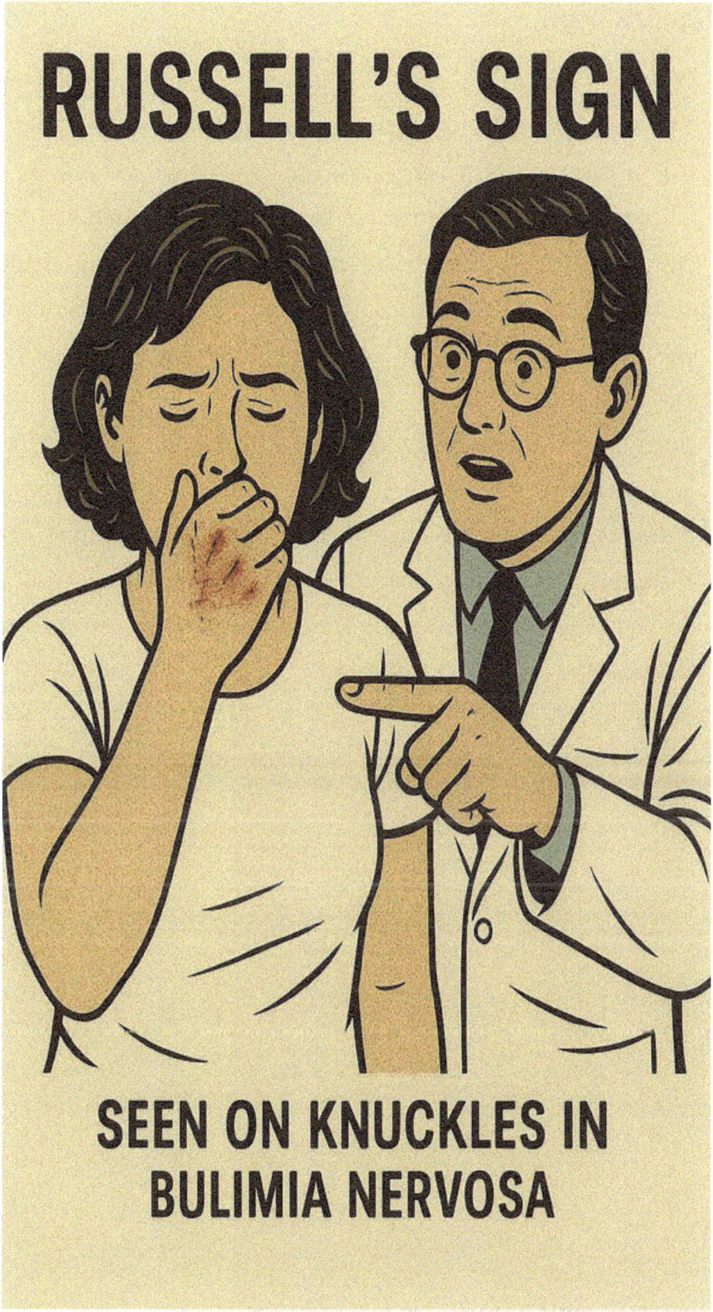
RUSSELL'S SIGN
SEEN ON KNUCKLES IN
BULIMIA NERVOSA

Rusell's Sign

- Named after the British psychiatrist Gerald Russell (1928-2018), this sign is observed in individuals with bulimia nervosa due to the recurrent contact of the incisors with the skin.
- This occurs during self-induced vomiting or when triggering the gag reflex by using their fingers at the back of the throat.
- It refers to the lacerations, abrasions, and callouses seen on the back of the hand, affecting the metacarpophalangeal and interphalangeal joints.
- Such scarring is recognized as one of the physical signs linked to a mental health condition.
- Russell's sign is mainly identified in those suffering from eating disorders like bulimia nervosa or anorexia nervosa.
- Nevertheless, it is not always a dependable sign of an eating disorder.

TREATMENT

Category	Details
Seen In	• Eating disorders, especially bulimia nervosa — repeated self-induced vomiting causes trauma to the dorsum of the hand (knuckle calluses)
Diagnosis	• Physical examination: calluses/ abrasions on knuckles- Psychiatric and nutritional evaluation for bulimia
Primary Treatment	• Multidisciplinary management:- Psychotherapy (CBT)- Nutritional rehabilitation- Psychiatric care for underlying eating disorder
Adjunct Care	• Skin care for hand trauma- Treat dental erosion, electrolyte imbalances, and other systemic effects
Follow-Up	• Ongoing psychiatric follow-up and medical monitoring are essential

Pathognomia

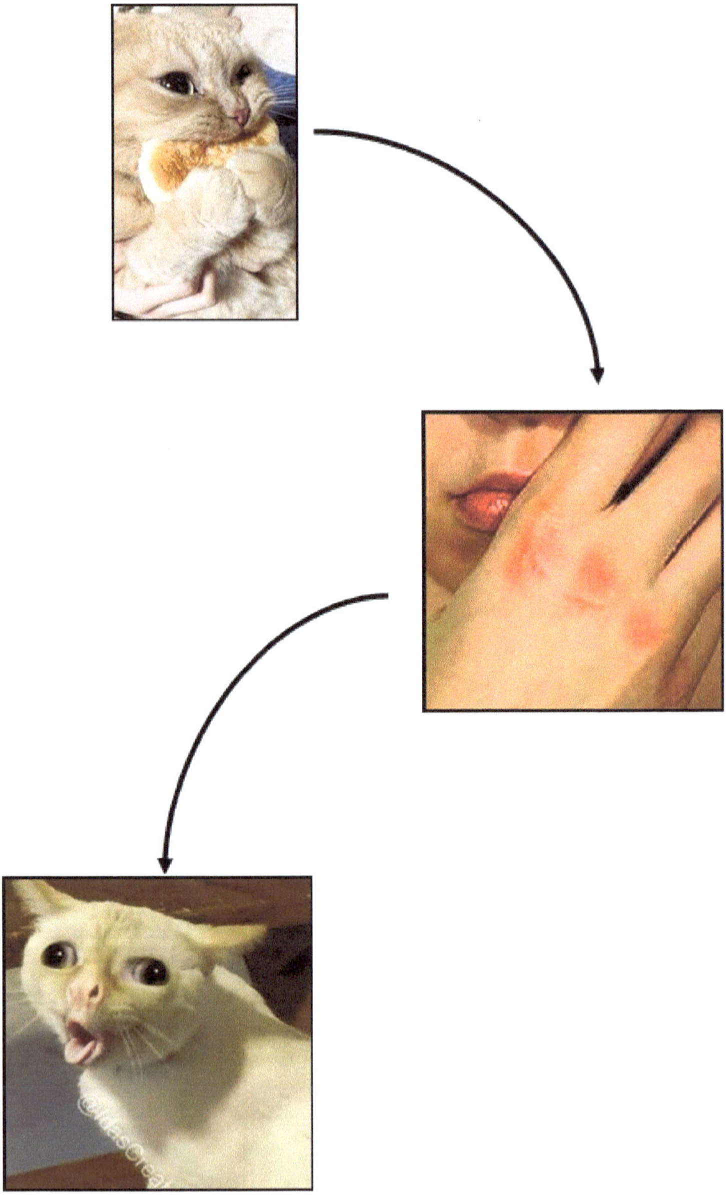

Allison Nitsch, MD, Heather Dlugosz, MD, Dennis Gibson, MD and
Philip S. Mehler, MD, FACP, FAED

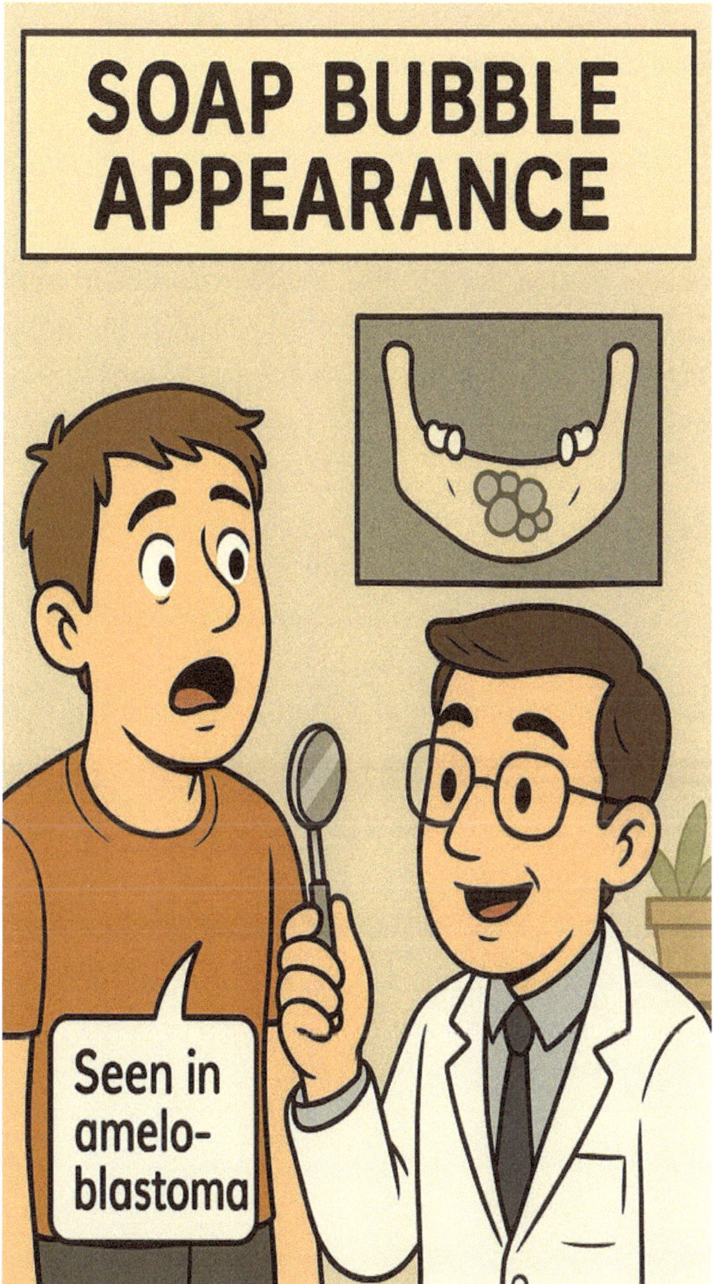
SOAP BUBBLE
APPEARANCE
Seen in ameloblastoma

Soap Bubble Appearance

- It describes a radiological appearance that has multiple compartments.
- **Radiographic features**
  In the skeleton, "soap bubble" is used to describe an expansile lytic bone lesion with internal trabeculations and preserved cortex, usually of benign nature but may be used to describe more aggressive lesions.
- **Differential diagnosis**
  - **Bone**
    - Aneurysmal bone cyst (ABC)
    - Giant cell tumour (osteoclastoma)
    - Adamantinoma of the jaw (ameloblastoma)
    - Plasmacytoma
    - Fibrous dysplasia
    - Chordoma
  - **Abdomen**
    - Meconium Ileus
  - **Brain**
    - Dysembryoplastic neuroepithelial tumour (DNET)
    - Multinodular and vacuolating neuronal tumour (MVNT)

Treatment

Category	Details
Seen In	• Ameloblastoma – a benign but locally aggressive jaw tumor
Diagnosis	• Clinical exam- Radiographs (soap bubble appearance)- Biopsy
Primary Treatment	• Surgical resection with wide margins (preferred to prevent recurrence)
Alternate Surgery	• Enucleation with curettage (higher recurrence risk)
Adjunct Therapy	• Not effective – chemotherapy and radiotherapy usually not indicated
Follow-Up	• Essential due to high recurrence rate

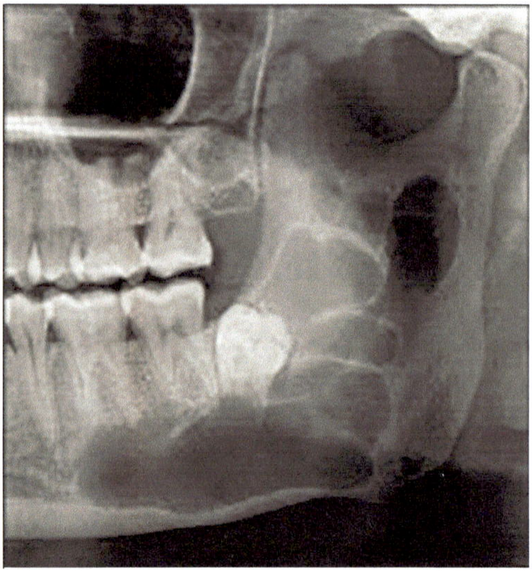

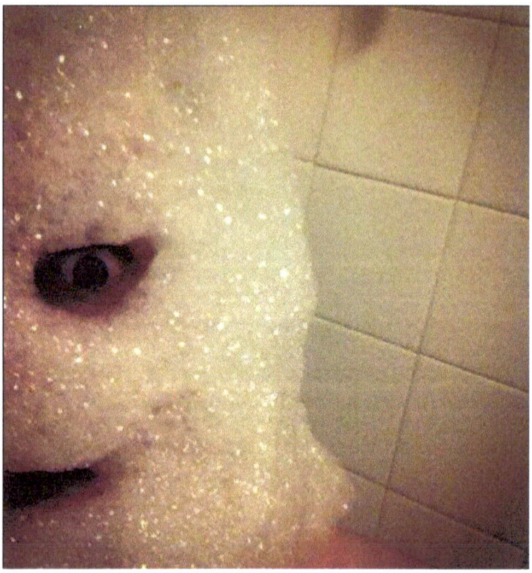

Phore, Swati & Panchal, RahulSingh & Baghla, Pallavi & Nabi, Nuzhat. (2015). Dental radiographic signs. Indian Journal 61 of Health Sciences. 8. 85. 10.4103/2349-5006.174234.

SECTION VI

REFERENCES

REFRENCES:

1. **Mutasim DF, Adams BB.** (2001). "The Asboe-Hansen sign revisited: Differentiating the blistering disorders." *Journal of the American Academy of Dermatology*, **44(4)**: 682–683.
2. **Schmidt, E., & Zillikens, D.** (2013). "Pemphigoid diseases." *The Lancet*, **381(9863)**: 320–332.
3. **Joly P, Horvath B, Patsatsi A, et al**: Updated S2K guidelines on the management of pemphigus vulgaris and foliaceus initiated by the European Academy of Dermatology and Venereology (EADV). *J Eur Acad Dermatol Venereol* 34(9):1900-1913, 2020. doi: 10.1111/jdv.16752
4. **Craythorne EE, Mufti G, DuVivier AW**: Rituximab used as a first- line single agent in the treatment of pemphigus vulgaris. *J Am Acad Dermatol* 65(5):1064–1065, 2011. doi: 10.1016/j.jaad.2010.06.033
5. **Nestle FO, Kaplan DH, Barker J.** (2009). "Psoriasis." *New England Journal of Medicine*, **361(5)**: 496–509.
6. **Menter A, Gottlieb A, Feldman SR, et al.** (2008). "Guidelines of care for the management of psoriasis and psoriatic arthritis." *Journal of the American Academy of Dermatology*, **58(5)**: 826–850.
7. **Kaur I, Saraswat A, Kumar B.** (2002). "A clinical and histopathological study of psoriasis." *Indian Journal of Dermatology, Venereology, and Leprology*, **68(6)**: 292–295.

8. **Dziurzynski K, Klie D, Riesenburger R, et al.** (2008). "Clinical and radiographic presentation of basilar skull fractures." *Journal of Trauma*, **65(2)**: 379–385.
9. **Rothrock, S. G., & Green, S. M.** (1997). "Basilar skull fracture: Does the Battle sign matter?" *Annals of Emergency Medicine*, **29(2)**: 223– 226.
10. **Friedman, J. H., & Factor, S. A.** (2000). "Tardive Dyskinesia: A Modern Overview." *Neurologic Clinics*, **18(1)**: 95–114.
11. **Correll, C. U., & Schulz, S. C.** (2004). "Oral Tardive Dyskinesia: Characterization and Treatment." *Journal of Clinical Psychiatry*, **65(Suppl 9)**: 27–32.
12. **Grossman ME, Fox LP.** (2003). "The 'carpet tack' sign in discoid lupus erythematosus." *Archives of Dermatology*, **139(4)**: 541–542.
13. **Khandpur, S., & Reddy, B. S. N.** (2005). "Discoid Lupus Erythematosus: A Clinical and Histopathological Study." *Indian Journal of Dermatology, Venereology and Leprology*, **71(4)**: 248–251.
14. **Cooper MS, Gittoes NJ.** (2008). "Diagnosis and management of hypocalcaemia." *BMJ*, **336(7656)**: 1298–1302.
15. **Rude RK.** (1998). "Hypocalcemia and neuromuscular irritability." *American Journal of Medicine*, **105(3)**: 296–303.

16. **Hartmann, K., et al.** (2016). "Cutaneous mastocytosis: Current perspectives." *Journal of Allergy and Clinical Immunology*, **137(1)**: 58–67.

17. **Tanno, L. K., et al.** (2018). "Mastocytosis: an updated practical overview." *European Annals of Allergy and Clinical Immunology*, **50(3)**: 108–118.

18. **Parapia, L. A., & Jackson, C. (2008).** "Ehlers–Danlos syndrome—a historical review." *British Journal of Haematology*, **141(1)**: 32–35.

19. **Grahame, R., Bird, H. A., & Child, A. (2000).** "The revised (Brighton 1998) criteria for the diagnosis of benign joint hypermobility syndrome (BJHS)." *Journal of Rheumatology*, **27(7)**: 1777–1779.

20. **Bell, R. B., & Dierks, E. J. (2005).** "Management of midface fractures."
Oral and Maxillofacial Surgery Clinics of North America, **17(1)**: 1–19.

21. **Abd-Elmeguid, A. (2010).** "Maxillofacial trauma." *Canadian Family Physician*, **56(12)**: 1295–1301.

22. **Zaal, M. J., et al. (2003).** "Risk factors for the development of chronic herpes zoster ophthalmicus." *Archives of Ophthalmology*, **121(2)**: 234–239.

23. **Kaufman, S. C., et al. (2000).** "Herpes zoster ophthalmicus: diagnosis, management, and prevention." *Cornea*, **19(5)**: 664–671.

24. **Gerwin, R. D., Shannon, S., Hong, C. Z., Hubbard, D., & Gevirtz,**
R. (1997). "Interrater reliability in myofascial trigger point examination." *Pain*, **69(1–2)**, 65–73.

25. **Simons, D. G. (2004).** "Review of enigmatic MTrPs as a common cause of enigmatic musculoskeletal pain and dysfunction." *Journal of Electromyography and Kinesiology*, **14(1)**, 95–107.
26. **Heymann, D. L. (Ed.). (2015).** *Control of Communicable Diseases Manual* (20th ed.). American Public Health Association.
27. **Rota, P. A., et al. (2016).** "Measles." *Nature Reviews Disease Primers*, **2**, Article number: 16049.
28. **Chaudhary, S., & Kumar, P.** (2023). Nikolsky Sign. In *StatPearls*. StatPearls Publishing. **Bolognia, J., Schaffer, J. V., & Cerroni, L. (2021).** ***Dermatology*** **(4th ed.). Elsevier. Habif, T. P.** (2015). *Clinical Dermatology* (6th ed.). Elsevier.
29. **Young, B. J., & Schultz, A.** (2023). Osler Nodes and Janeway Lesions.
30. **Baddour LM, et al.** Infective Endocarditis in Adults: Diagnosis, Antimicrobial Therapy, and Management. Circulation. 2015;132(15):1435–1486.
31. **Freiman, A., Kalia, S., & O'Brien, E. A.** (2006). *Dermatologic Signs.* Journal of Cutaneous Medicine and Surgery. CDC. (2024). *Symptoms of Scarlet Fever.* Retrieved from CDC.gov. *MedlinePlus.* (2024). Signs of scarlet fever.
32. **Bolognia JL, Schaffer JV, Cerroni L.** Dermatology. 4th ed. Elsevier; 2017.
33. **James WD, Berger TG, Elston DM. Andrews**' Diseases of the Skin: Clinical Dermatology. 13th ed. Elsevier; 2019
34. **Das, J. M., & Munakomi, S**. (2023). Raccoon Sign. In *StatPearls*. StatPearls Publishing.

35. **Herbella, F. A., et al**. (2001). "Raccoon eyes" (periorbital haematoma) as a sign of skull base fracture. *Injury*, 32(10), 745–747

36. **Russell, G. F. M.** (1979). *Bulimia nervosa: an ominous variant of anorexia nervosa. Psychological Medicine*, 9(3), 429–448.

37. **Manoharan, S. V. R. R., Behere, R. V., Praharaj, S. K., Kongasseri, S., & Sharma, P. S. V. N. (2014).** Russell's Sign in Persistent Delusional Disorder: A Case Report. The Journal of Neuropsychiatry and Clinical Neurosciences, 26(3).

38. **Sadock BJ, Sadock VA, Ruiz P. Kaplan and Sadock's** Synopsis of Psychiatry. 12th ed. Wolters Kluwer; 2021.

39. **Treasure J, Schmidt U, van Furth E**. Handbook of Eating Disorders. 2nd ed. Wiley; 2003.

40. **Balasubramanian, S., et al.** (2015). Aneurysmal Bone Cyst Secondary to Giant Cell Tumor of the Patella, *BMJ Case Reports.*

41. **Neville BW, Damm DD, Allen CM, Chi AC**. Oral and Maxillofacial Pathology. 4th ed. Elsevier; 2016.

42. **Marx RE, Stern D**. Oral and Maxillofacial Pathology: A Rationale for Diagnosis and Treatment. 2nd ed. Quintessence Publishing; 2012

43. **Das, A., Mandal, A., & Das, A. (**2021). *Splinter Hemorrhage of the Nail Bed: An Important Clue to Systemic Disease.* Cureus, 13(3), e13734.

44. **Habif TP.** Clinical Dermatology: A Color Guide to Diagnosis and Therapy. 6th ed. Elsevier; 2016.

45. **Kumar V, Abbas AK, Aster JC.** Robbins and Cotran Pathologic Basis of Disease. 10th ed. Elsevier; 2020.
46. **Taddio, A., Pellegrin, M. C., & Lepore, L.** (2020). *Kawasaki disease: The importance of prompt recognition and treatment.* Italian Journal of Pediatrics, 46, 146.
47. **Talha, B., & Swarnkar, S. A.** (2023). *Xerostomia.* In *StatPearls.* StatPearls Publishing.
48. **Auluck, A.** (2016). *How do I Manage a Patient with Xerostomia/Dry Mouth? Journal of the Canadian Dental Association*, **82**, g11.
49. **Chan AKY, Tamrakar M, Jiang CM, et al:** Clinical evidence for professionally applied fluoride therapy to prevent and arrest dental caries in older adults: A systematic review. J Dent 125:104273. doi: 10.1016/j.jdent.2022.104273
50. "NUG—Necrotizing Ulcerative Gingivitis: **A Review."** ***Journal of Community Medicine & Health Education.***
51. "Trench Mouth or Vincent's Angina**: A Noncontagious Anaerobic Infection."** ***Journal of Current Research in Scientific Medicine***.
52. *Vincent's Angina*. ***Pediatric Dentistry Open Access Journal,*** **7(4).**
doi:10.32474/IPDOAJ.2022.07.000268
53. **Langlais, Robert P., and Craig S. Miller**. Color Atlas of Common Oral Diseases. 4th ed. Philadelphia: Lippincott Williams & Wilkins, 2009.
54. **Wiegand, Susanne, et al**. "Vincent's Angina." Deustches Arzteblatt, 2 Dec. 2022,

55. **Sachdeva S, Sachdeva S, Kapoor P. (2011).** "Wickham striae: etiopathogenensis and clinical significance." *Indian Journal of Dermatology*, **56**(4), 442–443.

56. **Nandini AS, et al. (2022).** "A study of dermoscopic patterns of Wickham's striae in lichen planus." *International Journal of Research in Dermatology*, **8**(2), 206–211.

57. **Le Cleach L, Chosidow O**. Clinical practice. Lichen planus. N Engl J Med. 2012; 23;366(8):723–32. doi: 10.1056/NEJMcp1103641. Journal

58. **Weston G, Payette M**. Update on lichen planus and its clinical variants. Int J Womens Dermatol. 2015;1(3):140–149. doi: 10.1016/j.ijwd.2015.04.001. Journal

59. **Nandini AS, Zacharias M**. A study of dermoscopic patterns of Wickham's striae in lichen planus. Int J Res Dermatol 2022; 8:206-11.